D0250881

Success stories
from participants . .

"I've lost 43 lbs. and kept it off for a year. I fit into jeans my teenage daughter was hoping to wear. Oxycise! has been a life-saver at an extremely stressful time of life, and I realize for the first time in my life — I do have a choice in how I look and feel."

Trish Young, business manager

"After my 2nd child I kept putting on weight and feeling more lethargic. My doctor did some tests and discovered that I have virtually no thyroid function. He told me that it would be very difficult to lose weight with hypothyroidism. When I saw Oxycise! discussed in a magazine article, it made a lot of sense to me.

"I've lost 63 pounds, gone from a size 24 to size 14, and lost 6" from my waist and 10" from my hips. Oxycise! works and it's easy. I love that I can do it anywhere — in the car, while waiting for my children — I don't need a special spot. Truly anyone can do it!"

Karen Olive, mother of two

"I have literally spent thousands on diets and equipment, and didn't believe that breathing could help me lose weight. In only 14 days I lost 17 inches. After 60 days I lost 28 pounds and have gone down four dress sizes. Not only that, but I feel totally energized. It's a great program!"

Jane Ward, mortgage broker

"Oxycise! proved to be a very effective way to expend calories. In fact, the subjects burned 140% more calories with Oxycise! than riding a stationary bicycle. I can certainly see a variety of useful applications for Oxycise! — especially for those opposed to or unable to accomplish traditional exercise."

Dr. Robert Girandola, Ph.D., USC

"I am still amazed at the results I am getting. So far I've lost 45 inches! That is just incredible to me. But what is even more amazing to me is that I get up every morning looking forward to doing Oxycise! Thanks again for such an outstanding program and a great website!"

Heather Taylor

"My results were almost immediate. I was losing inches before I was even doing the full routine. Within seven weeks I reached my goal. I can now wear a bathing suit to our swim club and not feel like someone who just had a baby. I look and feel pretty darn good for being the mother of three children. Thanks to you, Jill, and to Oxycise!"

Taja Macconnell, mother of three

"I have multiple sclerosis and cannot do "traditional" exercises as I get very ill. I thought there was no hope until I heard of Oxycise! I was amazed! Not only was I capable of doing the program, I lost 30 pounds in the first two and a half months. I am absolutely thrilled!"
Jo Neuman

"I have moved my belt two notches in since last Monday. I am very pleased because I have had three lower back surgeries which left me with a leg limp, leg pain, and back pain. This is something I can do. Thank you!"
Rocco LaPenta

"It's absolutely unbelievable. Who would have thought that just by breathing I could get rid of the cellulite on my thighs that jogging three miles a day couldn't do."
Carla Hatz

"I simply don't recall a time in my life where I felt this good for this long. Not only have I changed my body from a size 16 to a size 10, I am in love with life again. Who would think that deep breathing for 15 minutes a day could have such a profound effect on a person?"
Lesleigh Hershkowitz

"The Oxycise! System is just too good to be true. I am down to 170 lbs. from 203 lbs. I feel like a celebrity with all of the attention I am getting from my co-workers. One of my residents met me about three months ago, and when she saw me last week she swore that I was not the same person she met earlier. I have just one word to say, THANKS!"
Mark Calloway, property manager

"I was depressed and desperate about my weight and had given up on any social life at college. I sought out your program and did everything you said. Within three months I lost a total of 40 pounds and 6 inches from my waist! I've maintained that for nearly a year without a lot of effort and can fit in pants I wore in 10th grade. In fact, a pair of shorts that I couldn't even pull up over my hips are now baggy! It is so fun to be able to hike and run and do other activities now. But the most exciting of all is I'm getting married next week! If I hadn't made these body changes, I would have never had the confidence to meet my new husband!"
Erin Gadd, college student

"I have spent many long hours crying myself to sleep, begging for a miracle by the morning. Nothing ever happened until you came into my life. Both my husband and my son can't believe the difference in just this short period of time. Now I can finally pay them back with a happier, healthier mom and wife. Please accept my sincerest and deepest thanks for making a miracle happen."
Gail Candline

"For the first time in over a decade I am totally medication free. I have not had any migraines for the two months I've done Oxycise! I have kissed my Prozac goodbye and have not taken any sleeping pills during this period. I cannot begin to express how good it feels to be free of those endless pills and to have so much energy.

"And by the way, I've lost five inches from my waist and two inches from my thighs. Thank you for putting me in touch with my body."

Vida

"I have not worn shorts in years and I went out yesterday and bought a couple pair of shorts. I have gone from pushing out of a size 16 to a size 10 and am so happy about this."

Joan Schofield

"Oxycise! has been the best investment of my life! I'm here to tell you that two weeks of Oxycise! has made more progress in my muscle tone and endurance than all the time I used to spend on the track and treadmill!!"

Machelle Wilbert

"I have dropped from a size 4 to a size 2 as well as dropped 4% off my body fat (17% to 13%). The great thing though, is that my lung capacity is so much greater now that my runs are much more enjoyable. Besides the weight loss and inch loss, the stress reduction benefits are so great that I had to write and thank you."

Debbie Secor

"I gained a lot of weight with my baby, and was so depressed that I couldn't get it off. Now, with Oxycise! I have gone from a very tight size 14 to a size 10. I am still losing more weight, and the last time I wore a jean size 10 was when I was a freshman in high school. I am smaller now than I was before I had my first baby!!!! Thank you so much."

Tera Brady

"I've suffered severe health problems and back problems for many years and have been so discouraged as I've gained so much weight. Now, for the first time in years, I can touch my toes easily, and my pants and skirts hang loosely. In the first two weeks I lost 3 inches off my waist. My back is stronger — even my chiropractor asked what I'm doing differently, because he noticed such a difference. Thank you."

Jerilee Hutchins, mother of two

"I am a 67-year-old voice teacher and when you get to be my age, everything slows down. Oxycise! is unbelievable! I lost 12 inches and five pounds in one month. Also my lower back has changed totally, in fact my massage therapist and chiropractor cannot believe the difference."

Winnie Hartman

"My wife and I both decided we needed to lose weight. She decided to buy a stationary bicycle, and I chose your program. After 7 weeks she hadn't made any noticeable change. On the other hand, I lost 3 ½ inches off my waist and 10 pounds. I feel good, and I have a smile on my face. I've introduced Oxycise! to several of my friends. You really have something here!"

Joseph Bishop, retired college president

"Jill Johnson's program is a lifestyle approach to fitness. It uses techniques that are easy to master, produce satisfying results, and can be incorporated into one's daily health and fitness. It combines isotonic muscle contraction with aerobic breathing to burn subcutaneous fat, increase heart performance, and strengthen major muscle groups.

"In three weeks I lost 1 3/4 inches off my waist. The muscle hardness in my abs is the same as when I do 400 situps a day. I am pleased with the results of the program and am incorporating much of it into my normal bodybuilding/training workouts."

Craig Kitchens, Utah state champion body builder

"Jill's seminars at Fitness Experience are extremely popular. She is a real inspiration to the participants in that she truly represents what she teaches.

"Many participants have finally found the exercise plan that works for them and their lifestyles through Oxycise! What I have seen is that people who are resistant to traditional exercise will actually do Oxycise! and receive the benefits. I highly recommend the Oxycise! plan for people who truly want to take care of themselves."

Jan McCasland, Evergreen, Colorado
Director, "A Fitness Experience"

"Since beginning Oxycise! I feel like I can breathe for the first time in years. I had used an inhaler four times a day to control my asthma, and now I find I don't need it at all!"

Jan Potter, Scottsdale, Arizona

"I've done aerobics, stretch and tone, and meditation, and always I felt dizzy with the heavy breathing (I have asthma). But Oxycise! is wonderful. I can easily fill my lungs and I feel more energized.

"I never dreamed I would meet you and find this wonderful way to take control of my body. Oh, thank you *so* much!"

Anne Roche, Boston, Massachusetts

"Oxycise! is almost too good to be true, because you expect things that are effective to be difficult — and this isn't. It's just a wonderful program."

Julie Gudmundsen, Vernal, Utah

For those who
truly seek health and joyful living.

My gratitude to everyone who has supported me through "thick and thin." A special thanks to my husband, without whom this book would have never been started — much less finished.

Also by Jill Johnson:

Books
Fuel for Success
Chart Your Success

Videos
Level One Video Set:
   Introduction to Oxycise! Basic Breath and Techniques
   Oxycise! Level One Workout
Oxycise! Level Two
Oxycise! Level Three
Oxycise! Level Four
Oxycise! Buns & Thighs I
Oxycise! Buns & Thighs II
Oxycise! Abs & Upper Body

Audiocassette or CD
Oxycise! On the Go Commuter Routine

For more information call
(303)224-9588

www.oxycise.com

Oxycise!®

Jill R. Johnson

Oxycise! International, Inc.
Conifer, CO

CAUTION!

The information contained in this book is not intended to replace medical consultation. The intent is only to offer health information to help you cooperate with your physician in your mutual quest for health. One should not participate in this exercise program, alter medications or change dietary habits except as advised by his or her physician.

Oxycise! International, Inc.
8170 S. University Blvd., #110
Littleton, CO 80122
(303)224-9588

http://www.oxycise.com

Cover by Karen Saunders
Photography by Joyce Jay
Illustrations by Karl Egbert

ISBN 1-890320-01-3

Library of Congress Catalog Number: 97-92981

Published in the United States of America

Oxycise! is a registered trademark of Jill R. Johnson.

Contents

Special Introduction

A Personal Letter to You

Dear friend who would love
to lose excess weight once and for all,

I have written this book for *you*. You are sick and tired of struggling with your body shape and health. You're angry at all the money you've spent and time you've wasted on pills, powdered drinks, and gadgets that promised to "save you." You're weary of missing out on opportunities because you don't have "the look."

Let's face it. Our society is absolutely obsessed with fat. How many times every day do you talk about it? How many times do you *think* about it? Whatever happened to discussions on politics, literature, or the arts? Now here's the kicker: How much money *and* time have you spent on weight loss products and weight loss schemes that have been useless? It's embarrassing.

Then there's the discrimination issue. The greatest discrimination that occurs in our country is not against minorities, but against people who are overweight, regardless of gender, sexual persuasion, or nationality. From the time we're infants, we're considered less capable, less intelligent, and less desirable if we carry excess weight.

And let's not forget the real health issues.

Here are some health facts[1]:

- When ideal weights for health are considered, it has been shown that 90% of women and 70% of men are overweight.

- Hypertension, high cholesterol, diabetes, and cancer (colon, rectum, prostate, gallbladder, breast, uterus, ovaries) are all considerably more prevalent in the obese compared to the nonobese. In the case of uterine cancer, the rate for women who are severely obese is 5½ times that of nonobese women.

- Extreme obesity is also associated with up to a 1,200% increase in death from all causes. And as men and women age, its death-dealing influence becomes more pronounced.

These numbers are scary! Have you been told to lose weight by your doctor? Have you been threatened by your doctor that you would experience serious medical complications (even death) if you didn't control your girth? I have. And I was only 27 years old at the time.

I recently met a woman who has some health problems that require a doctor's care, but she is way past due for her next doctor visit. Why? Because he hammered into her that she needed to lose weight to overcome those health problems. She hasn't lost the weight; and rather than face her doctor's displeasure, she's avoiding necessary medical care. Is there anything wrong with this picture?

Americans are so concerned with fat that $35 billion are spent every year on weight loss schemes and products. Can you imagine all the good that could be done in your home if that same money was channeled elsewhere?

Now before you get too discouraged, let me tell you the great news! There is a way for you and every other person to achieve an attractive, slender, healthy body.

I'm not talking about increasing your willpower. Dieters on the whole have so much willpower that many have tragically dieted themselves to death. Thousands of you continue to faithfully follow incredibly complicated and difficult regimens in your weight loss quest, never achieving permanent success. Many of you even cause damage to your body as you seek a svelte look.

Most of you are already expending more time and money than is necessary to achieve your goals, but there is one essential item missing:

Correct information . . . the right road map.

Oxycise! is the right road map for you to take control of your body! Remember, all your noble efforts at weight loss are worthless if you're following the wrong map.

So what can Oxycise! do for you?

---

1. Burn calories faster than traditional exercises!

In Chapter Three you'll see the results of studies done at major universities which dramatically show how much more effectively Oxycise! burns calories when compared to stationary bicycling.

---

2. Lose pounds and inches!

In a 15-minute session you can actually measure immediate results. Try it and you'll see!

---

3. Save time!

With most conventional exercise, you don't realize any results unless you spend several hours a week. With Oxycise! you can achieve fantastic results in only 15 minutes a day.

4. Save money!

My Personal Money-Saving Guarantee!

You will never need to buy another
weight loss pill, food, gadget, or product
if you follow the information in this book.

You will add hours to your week and dollars to your pocket because you won't have to:

- pay for expensive spa memberships.
- drive to the health club, change clothes, spend hours, shower, and clean up again.
- buy expensive equipment to take up space in your home.
- buy expensive shoes or workout outfits.
- arrange and pay for childcare while you walk for an hour every day.
- pay to attend "fat farms" for a week or more (using up vacation time and earning potential.)
- read the small print in all the newspaper and magazine ads claiming some new miracle cure.
- sit glued to an infomercial with pencil and paper in hand, ready to order the latest ab exerciser.
- pay obesity related healthcare costs.

5. Get rid of cellulite!

No more cottage cheese legs. You will stand amazed in front of the mirror.

6. Lower your set point weight!

You will literally change your metabolism and lower your set point weight. See Chapter Eight to learn more.

7. Improve your blood circulation and lower your resting heart rate![2]

Keep track of your resting heart rate as you add Oxycise! to your life and you will be pleased with the results. Also, as you get rid of extra fat and cleanse yourself of other toxins, you will remove unnecessary strain from your heart and provide a healthy blood supply for all your body systems.

8. Reshape your body!

No more spare-tire belly, saggy bottom, flapping arms, double chin, or fat cheeks.

9. Be stronger, last longer!

Listen to these unsolicited comments from Oxycise! clients:

"I feel so energized after a 15-minute workout!"

"I'm able to participate in my favorite recreational sports without getting winded or straining muscles."

"I am now able to breathe through my nose while I run."

"I've quit using my asthma inhaler."

"I don't take back pain medication any more."

"For the first time ever, I have nerve response in my damaged arm."

"I can join in with my kids at family activities."

"My back is stronger — even my chiropractor asked what I'm doing differently, because he noticed such a difference."

"I've been able to double my running mileage."

"I'm able to sustain notes longer when I sing."

Are you interested in any of the above benefits? All it takes is a small amount of the *right* kind of exercise to achieve the gorgeous, healthy body you deserve.

Oxygen is the key!

Oxycise! **is the answer!** It is extremely effective for men, women, and entire families of any age or fitness level. You can do it anywhere — home, office, motel room, or even outdoors. Oxycise! has even proven successful for those with back injuries, physical limitations, and disabilities.

These benefits are real! And you will start to receive them immediately. You will be transforming your body literally from the inside out. By using the amazing power of oxygen, you will be healing and nurturing your body starting at the cellular level.

How to get your money's worth from this book:

1.   ***Don't only read it once and put it aside. Do it!***

You, who want to look better and feel better than you ever have before, will do everything I tell you to do.

2.   ***Track your progress.***

This isn't a game. Do everything in this book as if your life depended on it, because it does.

3.   ***Share Oxycise! with a friend.***

You can do your part in freeing others from being slaves to their bodies. Join the crusade!

4.   ***Use Oxycise! to change your life.***

It will.

I am your personal trainer, your resource, your conscience, and your cheerleader. Do what I tell you to do. Learn the information and methods. You may get uncomfortable with some of the truths I share with you; but I don't like to live in a pretend world, so I'll be forcing you into reality once in awhile too. (Besides, what good does it do to continue to pretend you don't need to make some permanent body changes?) On the other hand, I will thrill with you in your successes.

I know first-hand the emotional pain of being fat and the physical pain of having a body that isn't healthy. Even more important, I know the wonderful freedom of having an attractive and healthy body. For over 10 years I have worked hard to research, document, and teach this amazing, yet simple, method that has become the basis for this book. It is now my mission, my crusade, to reach as many people as possible with these truths.

As you read Oxycise! and make it part of your daily life, I want you to imagine that I'm right there with you. I've learned that I don't have to physically be there with you for you to have success. In fact, one of the great things about Oxycise! is that you can personalize it to fit your schedule. I don't care how many failures you've experienced in your life, you will achieve success. *Oxycise! has a 100% success rate.*

I invite you to stay in touch with me. We are both still discovering and learning. After you've had some successes, I hope you'll contact me and share them. I know what you're going through. For this reason I want to be there to congratulate you as you succeed.

Implementing Oxycise! into your life will not merely benefit you personally . . . important as that is . . . it will also benefit everyone around you.

- Your spouse will love how you look.
- Your children will love that you have more time for them.
- Your boss will love your increased energy.
- Everyone around you will benefit from your increased vitality and joyful living.

Write me soon! I love to hear good news.

Your friend in health,

April 1997

8170 S. University Blvd., #110
Littleton, CO 80122
(303)224-9588

www.oxycise.com
email: jill@oxycise.com

Part One

The Problem

"All parts of the body which have a function, if used in moderation and exercised in labors in which each is accustomed, become thereby healthy, well-developed and age more slowly, but if unused they become liable to disease, defective in growth, and age quickly."

Hippocrates

Chapter One

Seventeen Reasons Why You Don't Have the Body You Want and Why You Will Never Have the Body You Want . . .

Unless You Oxycise!

In more than 20 years of working with people in different walks of life and on different parts of the globe, I have come in contact with many who have achieved tremendous success in some part of their lives such as business, family, personal character, or spirituality. And yet, these otherwise successful people have shared with me their pain, powerless feelings, and perceived lack of control in regard to their body weight and general health.

Perhaps some of their stories may sound familiar to you.

Personal Stories

"I bought a treadmill a year ago so I could exercise regardless of the weather. I used it faithfully the first month, but I didn't really notice many changes and I've gradually quit using it altogether. Every time I walk by it, I'm reminded of my lack of commitment. I'd love to get it out of my living room."

"I have tried every single food plan and pill that I see advertised, and yet I've never lost more than 10 or 15 pounds. I think I must have a thyroid problem."

"I work out for two hours every day; run several miles, lift weights, and play racquetball. I've kept this regimen up for many years and still my gut hangs over my belt and I have sizeable 'love handles'. What would happen if I stopped doing this?"

"It's impossible to lose weight when you're taking care of small children and a husband who demands dessert at every meal. I can't leave my children to go work out, and I don't have time to make my own special meals."

"I have a slow metabolism. It doesn't matter how little I eat, I cannot lose weight. All I have to do is look at that doughnut and it ends up on my thighs."

"I don't have time to count fat grams and calories, and I certainly don't have time to drive across town to the health club. If people don't love me the way I am then that's their problem."

"My husband harps at me all the time about my weight. Our physical relationship is nonexistent and I feel that he is disgusted with me. He's always suggesting I do some new weight loss program, but I've tried so many and I just keep gaining weight. It's hopeless."

"I would really love to focus my energy on something other than losing weight. It seems that it consumes so much of my time and attention. Isn't there something else I could be doing with my life besides struggling with my weight?"

These are real problems that will not be solved with quick-fix remedies. Before you can understand the principles in this book, you must first understand your own perceptions of taking care of your own body and health. Then you will be prepared to make the necessary shifts in the appropriate areas.

It is an established fact that the vast majority of people trying to lose weight or make any kind of body change not only fail miserably but often exacerbate the problem. According to *Consumer Reports*, those who lose weight by dieting gain it back within two years. Their survey of over 95,000 people included all the major dieting programs, including meal replacement shakes and even the more expensive programs that involve counseling and special foods. Most dieters also gain back considerably more weight than they lost during their diets.

Permanent weight loss is so rare that apparent "success" stories are featured on television talk shows. One major national program I saw recently had two women who had each lost over 100 pounds. I stayed tuned with interest to find out what their secrets were. The first lady had her stomach stapled. The second lady had gone through a major family trauma and severe depression leaving her without an appetite. Neither woman had yet been at that weight for one year, so the longevity of the weight loss is highly questionable. But more importantly, each woman had lost the weight with a very high risk of severe medical complications. Neither one had done it in a healthy way, and yet here was a famous talk show host complimenting them on their accomplishments.

I do not intend to let you be a failure at permanent weight loss or to let you lose weight while putting yourself at risk for other medical complications or problems. I intend for your efforts to be crowned with success — not just so you can fit into smaller jeans (delightful though that is) — but so you can achieve your optimum health and vitality, and so you and those around you can truly live life to its fullest.

This chapter sets forth the most common mistakes people make in weight loss efforts. You don't want to waste any more of your valuable time and money on mistakes. So read this chapter with pen in hand and commit to never making these errors. When you finish this and the following chapter, you'll know what *not* to do, and you'll have pledged not to ever do it again. As you read the rest of the book, you'll know just what *to* do, and you'll be well on your way to losing weight and gaining health.

The 17 errors that follow are divided into four related and yet distinct categories of mistakes. These four include the serious but avoidable mistakes of:

- *working against the laws of nature*

- *being influenced by the media*

- *thinking it's too hard*

- *poor breathing*

Remember, you must not merely identify with and understand these mistakes; you must not pretend that *you* have special powers, and that you can commit these mistakes and still have success. You must solve these problems. Your health, happiness, and slender body depend on it.

The

"working against

the laws of nature"

mistakes.

Avoidable Mistake #1
   You are following the wrong "road map."

You are conscientiously trying to make a body change. You
have a great attitude, lots of discipline, and no one could
fault you for will power. And yet, your body fat percentage
is still in the "poor" category, you are overweight, and nothing
you do seems to make any permanent difference. You feel like
giving up, but inherently you know that there must be a way to
bring your body into a healthy balance.

Most likely, you are simply following the wrong "map."
Somewhere along the line you have picked up a "map"
thinking it would help you reach your destination of a
healthy, slim body. Because you have been ineffective in
reaching that destination, you assumed it was your fault. So
you have worked on your behavior, discipline, and positive
attitude. You haven't arrived where you wanted, but you've
kept up your great attitude and perhaps even talked yourself
into believing it doesn't matter that you haven't reached
your destination.

The problem is you are still lost. You have not reached your destination and it has nothing to do with your behavior or attitude. It has everything to do with the fact that you have been following the wrong map. Most "maps" for weight loss should be titled "How to Temporarily Lose Weight and Then Gain It All Back Plus 10 Extra Pounds".

Oxycise! is the right road map. It is 100% effective and permanent. Once you learn and apply the correct principles described in this book, *then* diligence becomes important, and when you encounter frustrating obstacles along the way, *then* attitude can make a real difference. But the first and most important requirement is the accuracy of the map.

Right now you're making a decision. You've opened this book and as you read this paragraph, you are deciding your body size and level of health. You are the only person who has power over that. I will lay out an easy-to-follow map for you but you are the one who must follow it.

You *will* be able to achieve your dreams — losing 100 pounds or "those last 10 pounds," developing habits that will decrease your body fat percentage to a healthy level, decreasing as many clothing sizes as you desire, achieving body tone — by following the Oxycise! map.

Avoidable Mistake #2
> *You treat your body like a machine instead of like the incredible natural creation it truly is.*

If I see one more commercial selling a gadget or pill or chemical drink for weight loss, I'm going to scream!!! I mean, what are we??? Little machines? Do we need extra piles of metal in our homes, extra chemicals filling our cupboards? Okay, come clean. What do you have in your house? Just look around — Armmaster, Abmaster, Buttmaster, Thighmaster, Walkmaster, Runmaster, Ab Roller, Ab Rocker, resistance bands, weights, neoprene clothes . . . .

Open those cupboards! How many pills, gimmicks, gadgets, drinks, power bars do you have? And what's next to them? Oh yeah, chips, cookies, pop. Now the freezer, Lean Cuisine, Weight Watchers meals . . . and what's that?? . . . double-nut super-gooey fudge ripple ice cream?

What is going on? Who are you trying to kid? Is there any other animal on this earth that needs mechanical contrivances and chemically derived food to thrive? Are you any different?

Isn't it amazing
in our advanced age of scientific discovery,
so many people still struggle
with taking care of their bodies?

We live in an incredible time of high tech machines and chemically derived food. Have you forgotten that your body is natural? That is, it follows natural laws. *You cannot bypass these natural laws.*

Do you remember a time in your youth when your body served you? It did pretty much what you wanted it to do — skip, run, climb trees, jump rope, swim. You ate when you were hungry, stopped eating when you were full, smiled when you looked in the mirror . . . . What a carefree existence!

Have you become a slave to your body with addictions like drugs, nicotine, caffeine, fat, chocolate, sedentary living, and other choices that contradict health? The good news is if you really accept that your body follows natural laws and are willing to work within those laws, you will be thrilled to bring your body into your service again.

The goal of this book and the Oxycise! lifestyle is to bring you back in touch with your body so you may be *free* from obesity, addictions, and other physical ailments.   Never again will you feel the need to send in money for one more miracle drug, weight loss gadget, or appetite suppressant. Never again will you feel guilty because you didn't go out in a storm for your walk.

Oxycise! gives you the freedom to:

> Sit down without your stomach resting on your legs!
> Walk without your legs rubbing together!
> Bend over to tie your shoe without grunting!
> Climb a flight of stairs without gasping for air!
> Wave good-bye without your arm flapping!
> Sit on the beach without wearing a tent for a cover-up!
> Stand naked in front of a mirror and be proud!
> Try on new clothes and like how they look and feel!

If you like walking, running, cycling, or any other sports, you will have the health and energy to do them. But instead of forcing yourself to do these activities out of guilt, you will choose them for fun and pleasure.

No more will you be a slave to your body! You will master your body from deep inside because you have an influence on every cell in your body. That's the level at which you'll be operating. You will learn to call upon your own inner strength and power using your body's abundant natural resources.

**"The goal of life
is living in agreement with nature."**

Zeno, from Diogenes Laertius, VII, 87

Avoidable Mistake #3
You think your body has let you down and is not responding to your good care.

One cardinal rule in behavioral medicine is that unless it is interfered with, your body knows exactly what it is doing and always does the best thing it can do under the circumstances. Consequently, *if you are overweight, you may reasonably assume that the extra fat itself is your body's best adjustment to the circumstances you are providing.*

Contrary to what you may think, your body did not let you down. The extra fat is evidence that your body is doing the best it can with what is available. It makes sense, therefore, to ask, "What do I have to do to make it *un*necessary for my body to have to make this particular adjustment of storing extra fat?"

It's very possible that you have been following the wrong road map, as described in Mistake #1. Your body has been responding to whatever you've been doing to it. For instance, if you've been putting it through intermittent starvation exercises (a.k.a. dieting) then it's been taking good care of you by slowing down your metabolism and adding extra fat stores so it can last through those famines. You should be thanking your body, instead of giving up on it.

As you make Oxycise! part of your life, you will be thrilled and amazed at the changes you'll experience. You will not only feel better, but you will see visual changes occur that you thought were impossible. You will gain a sense of control and power as obesity becomes history.

Avoidable Mistake #4
   You use/consider food and sedentary living as rewards.

When you want to train your dog, one of the first things you do is get some dog biscuits or other treats to give your dog as rewards. You can literally get your dog to jump through hoops if you reward him with a little treat. Have you ever noticed how pervasive this same process is with humans?

"You've been such a good girl today, Mommy has a lollipop for you."

"If you finish everything on your plate you can have dessert."

"When you finish your chores you can choose a candy bar."

"You won the baseball game, let's treat the team to ice cream."

"I brought you this box of chocolates to let you know I appreciate your help."

"Our division had the highest production this quarter so the company is treating us to dinner."

"We worked so hard today, let's stop by the pastry shop for a treat."

I believe in giving rewards and positive reinforcement for a job well done, but can we raise ourselves a little higher than the dogs and give rewards that have longer-term benefits? How can a poor food choice be a true reward anyway?

Sedentary living has developed as another common "reward." If you've put in a hard week at the office in front of the computer, do you treat yourself to a relaxing weekend at home in front of the television? In our affluent times any task that requires physical movement is considered lower class, so in order to "treat" yourself you avoid physical exertion.

Stop it!

Switch your way of thinking. For a reward to be truly valuable it should have long term benefits. Yes, it's okay to take a nap on the couch or have ice cream once in awhile, but don't regularly use nonbeneficial items as rewards. Use a little creativity and think of what would really be a reward for a job well done. If you want to use food, then how about a fruit smoothie or other healthy choice?

Other rewards could be:

> Some extra time with your spouse or children.
> An evening with friends.
> A new pair of pants.
> A hike in the mountains.
> A day off for golf or skiing.
> Volunteer activities in your church or community.
> A bouquet of flowers.
> A facial.
> A massage.
> A bubble bath.

Choose something that is motivating and refreshing rather than "zoning out." Instead of giving children candy, try rewards like hugs, stickers, money, clothing, privileges, dates with mom or dad.

Giving your body a rest is very important when it is tired. But if it's really your brain or emotions that are tired, rejuvenate yourself with a walk, tennis game, bike ride, or Oxycise! As you feed your body more oxygen your metabolism will kick into action and you will not only nourish your body and feel more energy, you will also avoid gaining excess weight.

Avoidable Mistake #5
> *You embrace the Scarcity Mentality instead of the Abundance Mentality.*

When you look at a glass of water that is filled half way, do you describe it as "half empty" or "half full"?

Most people are deeply scripted in what has been termed the Scarcity Mentality.[3] They always view life, or any given area of life, in light of what is missing. They view life as having only so much, as though there were only one pie out there. And if they miss their share of the high-fat, high sugar foods and Lazy Boy reclining time, they feel deprived and robbed of their "piece of the pie."

Those with the Abundance Mentality, however, view life, or any given area of life, as an unending opportunity for growth. They thrive on and recognize the unlimited possibilities, options, alternatives, and creative solutions.

Here are some examples:

Scarcity Mentality

"I don't have time to pay attention to my body."

"If I spend 15 minutes a day on exercise then I'll have to drop my night class."

"I have to serve dessert or my children won't consider it a meal."

"There are so many yummy foods I'm missing."

Do you recognize any of these attitudes? Sometimes they are so subtle, we don't recognize how destructive they are. Now contrast the Scarcity Mentality attitude with the Abundance Mentality.

Abundance Mentality

"I gain so much time and energy by spending a few minutes each day on my body."

"There are so many benefits from living this lifestyle."

"I want to help those I love to enjoy good health."

"My friends and family are my allies in making the changes I desire."

As you continue to learn about and apply Oxycise! into your life, be sure and keep the Abundance Mentality in the forefront. Living a healthy lifestyle will only deprive you of poor health, lethargy, and fat. Living a healthy lifestyle will ensure that you have an abundant life with true benefits.

The

"being influenced

by the media"

mistakes.

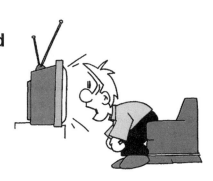

Avoidable Mistake #6
> *You're in search of the "quick fix" and "instant remedy."*

Over a hundred years ago, my great-grandpa came to Colorado to seek his fortune. He learned very quickly that all that glitters isn't gold. You've had your own experiences in seeking instant remedies for your weight problems just like my great-grandpa wanted an instant remedy for his financial problems. I'm going to guess you have had the same result as he did — a lot of money and effort spent with no measurable results.

It's easy to be drawn to the glitter of most other weight loss and exercise methods because of their sales pitches promoting some quick and easy way to achieve a trim body and good health without going through the body's natural processes. But "something for nothing" never has and never will work.

Fortunately with Oxycise! the results are measurable and immediate. By learning to harness your body's natural power you will be able to lose 2 to 4 inches from your waist during the first month. That's one pant size or more! You will lose inches from other body areas as well. As you consistently apply Oxycise! in your life, you will continue with a steady and permanent weight loss, as well as a dramatic decrease in body fat percentage of up to 5% or more in one month!

Avoidable Mistake #7
   Your mind has been imprinted with the need to diet.

Do you fit into any of these categories?

- You believe you can only lose weight if you limit your caloric intake.
- You follow any new diet that comes along.
- You have lost weight on a diet and gained the weight back.
- You use any form of appetite suppressant.
- You use weight loss drinks or liquid protein diets.
- You use weight loss pills.
- You use diuretics to lose weight.
- You have or are considering having your stomach stapled.
- You have or are considering having an intestinal bypass.
- You have or are considering having your jaws wired shut.
- You have done or are considering a medically supervised fasting program.
- You purge yourself with enemas or by vomiting.
- You are constantly dieting and are either getting fatter and fatter, or are destroying your health.

Stop it! Stop it now!

If you were alive during the 60s, 70s, 80s, and now the 90s, your mind has been imprinted with the need to diet. I get so angry at the continuous advertisements promoting appetite suppressants, diets, and limiting food intake in any form. Your appetite is natural. You are supposed to feel hungry so you will fuel your body when necessary. Surgically changing your body's digestive system is not only dangerous during the operation, but it keeps your body from doing what it is supposed to do. *Any* of the above listed actions keep your body from doing what it was designed to do. Altering these natural body systems and responses totally confuses and messes up your whole metabolic system.

Listen to your body. Right now close your eyes, take a deep breath, and relax. Visualize all the wonderful systems of your body . . . all the life force flowing through your veins and every single cell. Now visualize all 75 trillion cells choking, sputtering, and altogether misfunctioning because you are starving them. It's not a pretty sight. So just knock it off!

Due to the set point mechanism of your body, dieters depriving themselves of food — either through starvation or surgery — who succeed in losing weight initially will eventually gain it all back with a few extra pounds thrown in for good measure. Intermittently starving yourself is the most effective method available to add fat to your body.[4]

Please internalize this principle:

Dieting causes obesity.

A new Oxycise! convert, Julie Gudmundsen from Vernal, Utah, recently told me this story:

"I have a lot of friends who were losing weight taking appetite suppressants. They told me that I wouldn't have to go to any effort to lose weight because I wouldn't feel hungry and the pounds would come pouring off. I thought this was the answer for me.

"So I went to my doctor and got a prescription for the pills. I was actually taking the prescription at the time I read your book. I got to the section of the book that talks about setpoint and learned that dieting and pills play a trick on your body. I learned that when you stop dieting or taking diet pills, you will gain back the original weight and some additional pounds.

"I asked my doctor about this and he confirmed that when people stop taking diet pills, 99% of the time all weight will be regained, plus more. I didn't want that for me and I threw the pills away."

Stories like this really make my blood boil. How can doctors continue to knowingly prescribe pills that promote obesity and destroy their patients' health??? It's absurd!

Now just because I speak out on the evils of dieting doesn't mean you don't need to pay attention to what fuel you feed your body. On the contrary! You will be cleansing your body from the cellular level with Oxycise! so please don't muck it up with high fat food and dangerous chemicals. Be sure to spend plenty of time in the produce department at your grocery store and make food your ally in your quest for permanent weight loss.

Avoidable Mistake #8
> *You've been misled into believing that bouncing, shaking and sweating are the best ways to lose weight.*

For years the medical profession and fitness industry have shown that aerobic exercise, meaning exercise that increases your oxygen capacity, provides many benefits for our bodies, including weight loss. Somehow we have become accustomed to the idea that the only way to increase oxygen intake is by running, bouncing, dancing, and sweating.

Well, I would like to show you an amazing new way to increase your oxygen intake, boost your metabolism, and burn fat. Here's what you do:

> Breathe in.
> Breathe out.

Now do it with more intensity.

> Breathe in fully.
> Breathe out fully.

Did you injure your knees while you did that? Did you pull any muscles? Are you dripping with sweat? Did you hurt your back? Of course not!

You just made an important discovery!

Burning fat and increasing your oxygen capacity does not require ruining the rest of your body at the same time with hard impact exercise. In fact you don't need *any* impact. It does not require $80 shoes, or $1,000 spa memberships, or $200 exercise outfits. It does not require paying a babysitter while you work out. It does not require going out in bad weather, or having to shower and re-do your hair and makeup, or being annoyed by loud redundant music, or bright lights.

You are in for a treat as you do Oxycise! You can truly "rev up" your metabolism without bouncing, shaking, or sweating.

Avoidable Mistake #9
> *You've been sucked into trying to look like what the media presents as normal and healthy.*

This is typically a gender specific problem which overwhelmingly attacks teenage girls and women. Our society's current standard of beauty is an image that is literally just short of starvation for most women.

In his 25-year career, movie director Joel Schumacher has worked with, among others, Demi Moore, Julia Roberts and Sandra Bullock. But, he says, "I have never worked with a beautiful young woman who thought she was beautiful or thin enough. Sophia Loren and Marilyn Monroe could not get a job today; their agents would tell them, 'Go on a diet and get a trainer.'" He also says the teenage daughters of his friends are affected with eating disorders; one recently told him she belongs to a bulimia clique in her New Jersey high school. "I don't know what's going to happen to this generation of females," he says. "This obsession with being skinny is insane."

The definition of what constitutes beauty or even an acceptable body seems to become more inaccessible every year. Since 1979, Miss America contestants have become so skinny that the majority now are at least 15 percent below the recommended body weight for their height. (Medically, the same percentage is considered a possible symptom of anorexia nervosa.) In the past 30 years, the voluptuous size-12 image of Marilyn Monroe has given way to the size-2 bodies of current stars. The average height and weight of an American woman is 5 feet 4 inches at 142 pounds. Compare that to the average height and weight of current models, which is 5 feet 9 inches at 110 pounds, and it's easy to see why so many people feel dissatisfaction with their body size.[5]

Please remember that in order to have your body featured on the front of magazines, you have to devote your entire life to achieving that look. Many times, if not most of the time, it's only achievable at the expense of true health. Eating disorders, steroid use, and substance abuse run rampant in the entertainment industry.

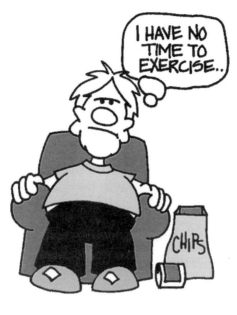

The

"thinking it's just too hard"

mistakes.

Avoidable Mistake #10
You don't have time to work out.

Don't feel alone. There are very few people who have a couple extra hours every day to drive to the club, change clothes, run a few laps, catch an aerobics class, lift weights, shower, dress, re-do hair, re-do makeup, and drive back to work or home. Of course you'd like to see your family once in awhile, maybe even do something around the house.

The fact is, even with all that time at the gym, you have a very slim chance of seeing any visual changes in your body. I continue to be amazed at the extreme amount of time necessary to accomplish body changes through traditional exercise methods.

Well you're in luck! Time will never be an issue with you again, because with Oxycise! you only need:

15 minutes a day!

With Oxycise! you will be able to make healthy and visual body changes in only 15 minutes a day. You don't even have to drive somewhere first before you start counting the 15 minutes. And the 15 minutes don't have to be consecutive.

All it takes is a small amount of the right kind of exercise to achieve the body you want. Oxycise! is the right kind of exercise.

Avoidable Mistake #11
  You don't want to spend hours reading treatises on exercise physiology.

You get bored reading the why's and wherefore's of how the body works. You want to get on with the process. That's just fine. The first part of this book is not required reading. Just skip it and go directly to Chapter Six and start to Oxycise! Or better yet, put the on video and get going.

Once you begin Oxycise!, you will never need to search out or read another book on weight loss.

Avoidable Mistake #12
You don't want to change any habits.

No one wants to change habits. Changing habits is hard, and besides, your body can still operate the remote. Why would you want to change anything?

More than likely you have made a lot of effort at some time in your life to change your habits in order to lose weight. You did everything you were "supposed" to do, but you didn't achieve permanent success. No wonder you don't want to change your current habits. It has never produced positive results in the past.

Your experience with changing habits is about to change. I'm not going to try and pretend that Oxycise! won't take any effort or habit changes. Changing direction always takes effort. But you're in luck! Your changes will be so well rewarded that you will hardly notice the effort.

Remember that it is gravity pull that keeps our world together, that keeps the planets in their orbits and our universe in order. It is a powerful force, and if you use it effectively, you can use the gravity pull of habit to keep you healthy and slender for a lifetime. Once you break out of the gravity pull of poor habits or mistaken habits, your freedom will take on a whole new dimension. The wonderful results will remain long after the discomfort of habit change has passed.

You are about to enter the Oxycise! orbit. Have courage to let go of things that aren't worth hanging on to.

Get ready for takeoff!

The

"poor breathing"

mistakes.

If you've ever suffered from asthma, or any respiratory problem, you know what it's like to crave oxygen. If you've ever had a boating accident or been pulled under water by an undertow, you know the desperation of being without oxygen.

Did you know that every single one of your 75 trillion cells needs oxygen in order to function at full capacity? That means your blood cells, your brain cells, your muscle cells, your vital organ cells . . . all of them!

Without oxygen you die! And it happens very quickly.

Just like you may have gasped for oxygen if you were caught under water or had something lodged in your throat, your cells may be "gasping" for oxygen all the time as you deprive them of this most essential nutrient in the normal course of your day.

I believe that most people who are overweight and unhealthy suffer from lack of oxygen. See if you do any of the following mistakes.

Avoidable Mistake #13
You are a shallow chest breather.

Chest breathing means you only expand the rib cage during breathing. Even though it may look more dramatic than diaphragmatic breathing, it is inefficient because only minimal air can enter and leave the lungs. You are basically only taking in enough air to survive but not enough to thrive.

The reasons for chest breathing are many: In trying to stay up with fashion you have cut off your oxygen intake by wearing tight pants, girdles, and belts. Perhaps you're required to sit at a desk all day in order to earn a living. Some of you may have developed panic disorders, asthma, or other respiratory problems.

Whatever the reason, if you are a chronic shallow breather, the obvious and immediate effect is poor ventilation of your lungs. This means that your body will have reduced levels of oxygen and your entire metabolism will be affected. Your body is trying to function in a primarily anaerobic state and you have set yourself up for a whole host of disorders including skin problems, heart disease, cancer, *and obesity.*[6]

Once again, let me emphasize this simple fact:

Your body needs oxygen
in order for every cell, tissue, and organ
to function correctly.

Stop looking for the magic pill that will solve your weight problem. You have the magic substance all around you — and it's free! Now it's up to you to capitalize on it.

Avoidable Mistake #14
You live in a push-button society.

Just think about life in times past. In order to survive, people had to move. From sun up to sun down, they had to keep moving if they wanted to live. There was hunting, plowing, taking care of animals, walking to get water, carrying water, scrubbing laundry by hand, beating the rugs, building your house, gathering wood, pushing, hauling, pulling, lifting, etc.

Today our society has become so automated that you can actually make a decent living virtually without moving. Many people are even working at a home office, so the farthest they walk is from one room to another, and the most they lift is the telephone to their ear. Others who still venture out in the cold, cruel world may have a few more physical requirements:

> walk to the car in the garage
> push the garage door opener
> punch in the code at the car wash
> order food at the drive up window
> push in the numbers at the ATM machine
> stick in the card at the parking garage
> walk through the automated doors
> push the button on the elevator
> walk to the desk
> sit down at the computer and . . .

> You get the picture!

Of course, there are still a few jobs that do require physical exertion, but they are becoming less common. I'm not saying buttons and machines are bad. I love not gathering wood and cooking over a fire every day. *But our breath has become shallow.* Our daily physical activities do not guarantee that we will breathe deeply and deliver the optimum amount of oxygen to our cells. The result is not only obesity but poor health and body malfunction.

It's wonderful to live with all of our modern conveniences, but you must breathe deeply and well. As I teach Oxycise! to people around the country, I always receive such enthusiastic comments from people experiencing instant and significant responses in their bodies by simply improving and increasing their breathing. It's really true that the best things in life are free!

Avoidable Mistake #15
   Stress has literally "taken your breath away."

Even though we have so many labor-saving devices, somehow our culture has developed such a high production mode that instead of enjoying the benefits of technology, we have increased demands and expectations. Stress has become a major health issue.[7]   With stress, fear, anxiety, and pressure, once again your breathing is altered.

What's the first thing that happens when you feel anxious? Your breath pattern changes, doesn't it? Have you ever been so tense that you could barely breathe? Your chest feels constricted and you gasp for air? Or perhaps you even hyperventilate?

If you limit your breathing with short, shallow breaths, what do you think happens to the rest of your body? Your cells cannot operate. Everything from your brain, heart, digestive system, and every other body system is deprived of its most essential nutrient. When stress sends the triglyceride levels up in the blood, clumping and sludging of the red cells occurs. This clogs up the capillaries and interferes with oxygen delivery by the red blood cells.[8]

In addition to lethargy, weak muscles, and a host of diseases, your body's metabolism is thrown off balance. An extremely common result is weight gain. Your body just doesn't have enough oxygen to cleanse itself properly and metabolize cells for nutrients.

I experienced this problem personally a couple years ago. Now keep in mind that I already had incorporated Oxycise! into my life and had been healthy and slender for several years. My family went through an extremely difficult trauma and I responded with breathing problems. As I worried and dealt with this trauma my breathing became more and more restricted to the point that I couldn't sleep well at night. I would lie there and try to relax my body so that I could get enough oxygen in. Over the course of the year I gained 20 pounds and had to buy pants two sizes bigger. That was depressing. Previous to that episode, I was confident in my ability to stay in touch with my body. But I learned that I still have more experiences to go through.

The good news is that when I finally realized what was happening to my body, all I had to do was reincorporate the Oxycise! principles I already knew. Within six weeks I lost the 20 pounds and fit back into my normal clothes. Not only that, but my general health was greatly improved, as well as my stamina and strength. My only regret is that I neglected to use the principles I knew at a time when I needed them most.

I won't attempt in this book to address how to emotionally deal with any stress, fear or anxiety you may be facing. However, I guarantee that if you keep your breathing deep and strong, doing the things you will learn in Oxycise!, your body will not fail you in your time of need. In fact, very likely it will become the healthiest and strongest it has ever been, and you will be in a better position to cope with and solve external pressures.

Avoidable Mistake #16
   You don't eat oxygen rich food.

In our instant, prepackaged, fast-food society you have sacrificed health for instant foods. You realize you need to breathe in oxygen, but you have neglected the other major source of oxygen — eating fresh food.

The home-prepared meal or the *good* restaurant foods you look forward to at the end of the day are oxygen depleted because they are mostly cooked. This means no oxygen or enzymes remain to help you digest and assimilate the meal. Cooking (heating) fruits and vegetables and roasting nuts and seeds drives out oxygen. Not only are hydrogenated and processed foods oxygen poor, they add a lot of debris (indigestible food particles) that overtax the already overworked circulation system. It requires time and effort for the body to haul this debris around in the bloodstream, leaving less time and energy for the body to take in oxygen. The result is oxygen deficiency.[9]

Even though you're putting some kind of food in your body, you probably suffer from cravings. If you try to satisfy those cravings by giving your body even more dead, overcooked, greasy, artificially colored, artificially flavored, saturated-with-preservatives food, then you will never feel satisfied even though you are physically stuffed. *And* you've actually starved your body of essential nutrients, especially oxygen. Overeating of oxygen-poor, nutrient-deficient, cooked and processed food is a slow, torturous death.[10]

Avoidable Mistake #17
You don't Oxycise!

This is the ultimate avoidable mistake! Prior to now you had an excuse, you didn't have the information — the right road map. But now you have it right in your hands and if you don't use it, then you are responsible for not having the body you deserve. Remember that having these tools and not using them makes you no better off than you were without the tools.

Oxycise! follows natural laws and achieves permanent results. You have in your hands the road map to success. Remember you cannot fail with Oxycise! It is a lifestyle not a temporary program.

You are going to love it!

Chapter Two

Thirty-Six Reasons Why Other Programs, Products, and Methods Fail to Help you Lose Weight

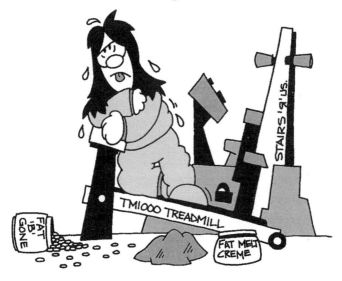

You've tried every method, every diet plan, every pill, every machine and you still don't have the body you want. You feel like a failure. If something is advertised on TV, or in a magazine, or recommended by your doctor, doesn't that mean it will work as long as you have self-discipline? *You just must not have any willpower.*

Cut! Stop the tape! You *do* have determination, willpower and a positive attitude. **What you haven't had is the right road map.**

Now before I present the right road map in its entirety, I want you to understand the limitations of the common programs, products, and methods currently advertised. Although some are not inherently harmful, they do not encompass all the components you need to achieve your goals permanently.

The problems with *"food emphasis"* programs, products, and methods.

Food emphasis programs, products, and methods include the likes of Weight Watchers, Jenny Craig, Slimfast, Acutrim, Medifast, Optifast, diet pills, appetite suppressants in any form, meal replacement shakes, "metabolism changing" pills, any fasting or starvation program, stomach stapling, intestinal bypass, jaws wired shut, diuretics, purging, etc.

1. These are all based on the errant philosophy that overeating is the cause of weight problems.
2. Many of these rely on weighing or measuring food which promotes feelings of "diet" or deprivation.
3. Many have you rely on and purchase their special foods or chemicals, preventing you from learning to utilize fresh, natural, healthy, and easily accessible food.
4. Impossible and unhealthy to maintain for a long period of time.
5. There is little or no physical activity promoted.
6. Your metabolism typically slows down dramatically causing lethargy and other physical problems.
7. Dieting is one of the most effective ways to *gain* weight.

8. They only provide short-term approaches, rather than a permanent lifestyle.
9. You are loading your body with chemical overdoses.
10. They often promote psychological issues with food.
11. They do not increase oxygen capacity and consumption.
12. They are usually very expensive.
13. Many of these put you at risk of severe medical complications — even death.

The problems with *"mind emphasis"* programs, products, and methods.

These include hypnosis, motivational tapes, motivational talks, motivational groups, books, etc.

14. These usually focus on willpower and determination leaving out the biggest cause of failure: *Following the wrong road map.*
15. They operate with the erroneous concept that overweight people lack discipline and willpower.

The problems with *"gadget emphasis"* programs, products, and methods.

These include treadmills, rowing machines, stair machines, cross-country ski machines, Ab Cruncher, Ab Roller, Thighmaster, resistance bands, weights and barbells, etc.

Anything that promotes safe movement is not harmful, but these products are not the most productive in losing weight.

16.   Most of these are very expensive.

17.   They take up space in your living room or bedroom.

18.   They don't address nutrition.

19.   They don't provide measurable results in a reasonable amount of time.

20.   None of them work the entire body simultaneously.

21.   Not conveniently transportable, you have to purchase machines or join a health club.

22.   When traveling or during inclement weather, they are difficult to keep doing.

23.   Not usable by all ages and fitness levels.

24.   With a machine at home only one person at a time can use it, causing scheduling problems.

25.   Because measurable changes take so much time and effort, most people are unable to maintain this kind of time commitment.

The problems with
"traditional exercise"
programs, products, and methods.

These include aerobics classes (high impact, low impact, step, slide), jogging, walking, calisthenics, swimming, water aerobics, bicycling, etc.

26.   They don't address nutrition.

27.   Overweight or nonathletic people rarely participate.

28.   With most of these you have to leave your home or office, which then introduces other problems:

weather, child care, club membership costs, scheduling, changing clothes and showering two or three times a day, etc.

29. Many injuries occur — knees, back, shin splints, feet problems — most of which become permanent. A participant at one of my workshops recently told me how she had attended aerobics classes until her zealous instructor pushed her to jump and kick higher, and she fell on her tailbone and fractured a vertabrae.

30. Heavy sweating makes it difficult to do this type of exercise between other activities.

31. There is little or no flexibility development.

32. You need special shoes and clothing.

33. Body changes take an extreme amount of time.

34. Many muscle groups are ignored, especially the abdominal area.

35. You have to schedule your life around the class time.

36. There is a major time investment.

No wonder you haven't been successful
with these programs!

How disheartening to have put so much effort into ineffective processes. Now I want you to compare the above problems with the benefits of Oxycise! listed in the next chapter.

By making Oxycise! part of your life, you will achieve success once and for all!

Part Two

The Cure

"The doctor of the future will give no medicine, but instead will interest his patients in the care of the human frame, in diet, and in the cause and prevention of disease."

Thomas Edison

Chapter Three

Oxycise!

Is the Answer

Oxycise! is about POWER!
　　. . . the power each of us has within to live a life of joy.

With Oxycise! you will experience JOY!!! The joy of being
slender and healthy. The joy of being free to choose the best
fuel for your body and the activities that will keep your
body full of vitality. You will be amazed at how simple it is
to accomplish these things. I have been able to accomplish
it and I'm just a normal human, living in a normal house
with hubby and kids. I do normal things like work, go to
church, make regular trips to the grocery store, take kids
to piano lessons and baseball games, go to parent/teacher
conferences, clean toilets, and do laundry.

Having power over your body is within the reach of every
person who can breathe and think! You want to come to
grips with your health once and for all, and *this is the right
book* to help you. You have the power to have a trim, healthy
body without machines or chemical food substitutes.

University study demonstrates the power of Oxycise!

Studies have been done at major universities to explore the caloric expenditure and oxygen consumption of Oxycise! The most recent was at the University of Southern California in May 1996. Gas analyzation equipment was used to measure the caloric cost of Oxycise! and to compare Oxycise! with a traditional form of exercise, namely a stationary bicycle. This study did not explore all the ramifications of the Oxycise! program but was intended to indicate whether the caloric expenditure and oxygen consumption were comparable to exercise on a stationary bicycle.

The results were dramatic! Here are the comments of the director of the testing, Dr. Girandola:

"In terms of weight control, the key goal is to try to increase your caloric expenditure, and any way you can do that has got to be beneficial. What we found was that Oxycise! was approximately four times resting metabolic rate. In addition, we had two subjects pedal a bicycle unloaded and found that in both subjects, the caloric cost of Oxycise! was 140% higher.

Oxycise! burns 140% more calories than riding a stationary bicycle.

"Now this is very surprising to me, that by just doing a breathing exercise someone could achieve that kind of caloric expenditure. Many people who don't like to exercise, or don't find time for it can benefit from this program."[11]

You should also note that in order for bicycling to utilize this much oxygen or burn this amount of calories, it is necessary to warm up first. With Oxycise! the results are immediate and can be done intermittently throughout the day without any warm up.

Another major difference is that everyone can do Oxycise! If you've ever tried to ride a bike for an extended time, you know that it's extremely difficult and you will be left dripping with sweat. In addition, only the legs are exercised in a forward motion while the rest of the body just sits there on the hard seat.

It's true! If you have given away control of your body, with Oxycise! you will have the power to reclaim it.

What Oxycise! will do for you.

1.   Burn calories faster than conventional exercise.
2.   Increase metabolism around the clock.
3.   Get rid of fat and cellulite.
4.   Lose weight.
5.   Lose inches.
6.   Lower your set point.
7.   Build lean body mass.
8.   Lower your body fat percentage.
9.   Reshape your abdomen, thighs, buttocks, legs, arms, face, and neck.
10.   Increase endurance.
11.   Increase strength.
12.   Increase flexibility.
13.   Save time.
14.   Save money.

15.   Reduce stress.
16.   Improve energy level.
17.   Improve alertness.
18.   Strengthen back and spine.
19.   Orthopedically beneficial.
20.   Improve skin tone.
21.   Maximize oxygen consumption.
22.   Improve blood circulation.
23.   Improve digestion and elimination.
24.   See and feel results within the first week!
25.   Bring your body shape and weight into a healthy balance.

One of the most appealing aspects of Oxycise! is that you can do it in the privacy of your own home. It's easy to do in a motel room, your office, or even in your car.

And it's safe! Oxycise! is safe for people of all ages and fitness levels. You don't ever have to worry about twisted ankles, pulled muscles or shin splints, side effects from chemicals, or any other side effect from traditional weight loss methods.

I'll close this chapter with the words of Dr. Mark Akers, a chiropractor in Colorado who recommends Oxycise! to his patients.

"If you want to decrease stress, increase your mental acuity, decrease blood pressure, lose inches and pounds, then I highly recommend the Oxycise! program for you."[12]

Chapter Four

I Breathe, Therefore I Am

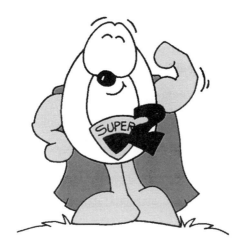

The Power of Oxygen

Your body needs three main fuels:

Food

Water

Oxygen

What's the Number One Body Fuel? You guessed it,

Oxygen!

How basic can you get? From the time we were little kids, we knew we needed oxygen to stay alive. We learned not to put plastic bags over our heads and not to play hide and seek in refrigerators. Some of us even tried to control parents by holding our breath. But if our bodies have developed somewhat normally, we have taken breathing and oxygen for granted.

How many of you breathe on a regular basis? When was the last time you thought about it? Aren't our bodies wonderful? They just keep on working and working without much thought from us. . . or should I say, in spite of us!

It seems to be only in times of crisis (heart attack, upcoming class reunion, etc.) that we make any effort to improve ourselves. And then, when we have done enough to "get by", we go back to our former harmful habits and ignore our bodies until the next crisis (wedding, swimsuit season, second heart attack).

Remember that if you are overweight, your body did not let you down. The excess fat is evidence that your body is doing the best it can with what is available.

Now I want you
to lean
real close,
'cause I have a secret
to tell you . . .

Breathing is the key!

Breathing is the key that unlocks the power of your body to achieve its full potential. It is the first step on your journey to a slender, fit body.

It's the King!

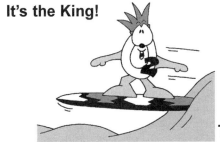

The Big Kahuna!

Do not take this lightly!! Breathing is life! It is the way to achieve vitality and joyful living!

Do you know what happens every time you breathe? When you inhale, the air enters in through your nose or mouth and continues down through your windpipe (trachea) into your lungs. The trachea branches into two bronchi, which then rapidly divide into a branching mass of smaller air tubes called bronchioles, and then into the small clusters of alveoli (air sacs). This is where gas exchange takes place.

Interesting fact:

> If all the alveoli from both lungs were opened up and laid flat, they would cover a tennis court.[13]

The microscopically thin wall of the alveolus and the blood vessel are fused together to form the respiratory membrane.

Oxygen from the alveolus passes into the blood, flows from the lungs, through the left side of your heart, to the body tissues. The blood delivers oxygen to every cell and picks up carbon dioxide. It then returns through the right side of your heart to the lungs, and the carbon dioxide from the blood passes into the alveolus by diffusion. This gas exchange process occurs rapidly and continuously.

Aren't our bodies amazing? And we don't even have to think about all this while it's happening.

What does this mean to you?

Oxygen helps your cells metabolize nutrients for energy, maintenance, repair, and healing. The way you breathe has a profound effect on your heart, arteries, and blood flow. Breathing affects the diameter of your blood vessels, your blood pressure, and the work output of the heart. The activity of your brain is directly affected by the way you breathe.[14]

Chief body cleanser.

Breathing is also your chief body cleanser. Elimination of wastes, debris, toxins, and body pollution is a major function of oxygen.[15] Do you realize that much of your body's waste is eliminated through exhaling? In fact, carbon dioxide is the most abundant of all the end-products of metabolism.[16] (The rest of your waste is eliminated through urine, bowels, and perspiration.) When your body can't eliminate properly, it stores the toxins and you have to live with them all the time. How does that extra poundage feel?

Using cameras inside the body, J.W. Shields, MD, found that deep, diaphragmatic breathing stimulates the cleansing of the lymph system by creating a vacuum effect which pulls the lymph through the bloodstream. This increases the rate of toxic elimination by as much as 15 times the normal rate.[17]

So if you limit your breathing, your body is deprived of the oxygen it needs to cleanse itself. Not fully utilizing the oxygen available to us has created the large toxic "waist" dump with which our nation's environmentalists should be most concerned.

By reading this are you starting to breathe more deeply?
GREAT!
Doesn't it feel good?

Now it's time for another secret. I've already shared some secrets with you, but this one is my personal favorite . . .

Fat leaves your body through carbon dioxide.

It does not dissolve with "magic" pills and come out in your urine. It does not melt away into sweat under neoprene shorts or waist belts. It does not disappear by smearing creams on your thighs or lounging in vibrator belts. And it does not disappear through wishful thinking.

Fat is the only one of the three major classes of food material that is stored free of water. Carbohydrate and protein are stored in combination with water, which forms more than half the total weight of these stored materials.[18] So if you think diuretics are a cure for fat, think again.

> Note: By the way, don't deprive yourself of water. The amount of water in your body is an important factor in muscle growth because protein synthesis takes place in the presence of water. That means that if you want to promote muscle growth (and muscles burn lots of calories) drink plenty of water.[19]

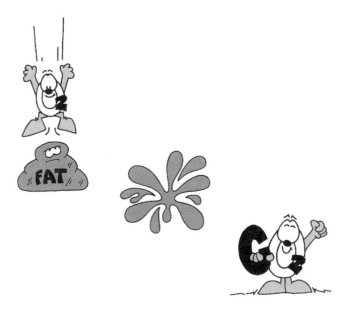

Fat is made up of atoms of carbon, hydrogen, and oxygen.[20] When you breathe and take in oxygen, the fat molecules are combined with the additional oxygen atoms causing oxidation. The products are carbon dioxide (made up of atoms of oxygen and carbon) and water (made up of atoms of oxygen and hydrogen).[21]

This is a BIG DEAL!

Does this information give you any ideas?

Let's see, hmmm. . . .

> "Fat leaves my body through carbon dioxide."

> "I can increase my capacity for oxygen/carbon dioxide exchange by breathing more deeply."

> "That means — voila! — *I can burn extra fat with increased deep breathing!"*

> "Why didn't I ever think of this before?"

Although breathing is automatic, it is also the *only* vital life function that you can voluntarily control. (Did you ever try to tell your heart to stop beating or your stomach to stop digesting?) Therefore you can actually affect your metabolism.

This means that by increasing oxygen, you can bring your own body's metabolic process into balance.[22] It means that your body will fully cleanse itself at the cellular level, releasing toxins that result in health problems, *including obesity.*

Remember that your body will always do the best it can with what you give it. Why not give it more?

Oxygen is FREE!

Oxygen is easy to increase.

Oxygen doesn't take up extra room in your living room or medicine cabinet.

You can find oxygen in all parts of the world.

You don't have to wait for the FDA to approve it.

No prescription is necessary.

There's plenty of it.

You never run out.

Side effects.

As with everything you take into your body, there are definite side effects, so study this list carefully to be sure you won't have any results that will be detrimental to your current lifestyle.

Effective weight loss

Lower set point weight

No more cellulite

Increased alertness

Reduced stress

Increased athletic performance

Better skin tone

Improved sexual response

Improved blood circulation

Better digestion and elimination

Deep, relaxing sleep

Vibrant health

I don't know, it's a tough call . . .

hmmm, I think I'll choose breathing.

Chapter Five

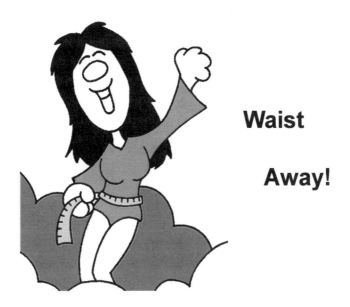

Waist

Away!

Medical experts now claim that the biggest health concern in our society is "waist circumference."[23]   In other words, having extra fat around your middle is a BIG health problem and not just an appearance problem. All your vital organs are in your trunk area, so if you carry extra fat there, you are suffocating those organs and preventing them from functioning well.

It's amazing to me how much this part of the body is neglected in conventional exercise these days.   One would think that our legs (quadriceps) are the life-giving core of our entire being. What little attention is given to the trunk area is in the form of crunches and situps. Doesn't it occur to anyone that all our vital organs are here? If we build support and strength in this area and increase oxygen and circulation here, all of our extremities will benefit.

How do you get rid of your gut?

Nearly every magazine you pick up has some promise of "Great Abs in Five Days," or something similar. If you turn to the article it will once again describe and show pictures of some variation of the good ol' situp, crunch, or leg lift. On TV there are gadgets advertised that are more variations of the crunch — only some claim to prevent damage to your back. Do *you* personally know anyone who has made a substantial change in their "waist circumference" by doing these exercises? I don't.

The truth is, anyone who has more than a couple inches to lose off their abs will have an extremely difficult time doing those types of exercises, and it will be doubtful if they will stick with them. In addition, there's a high risk of injury and a low possibility of significant results. And what about the millions of us who have back injuries, which means that putting pressure on our spine in that manner would be extremely painful and damaging?

Much research has proven what us regular people have discovered on our own:

> "Traditional sit-ups and leg-lifts don't slim the waistline, no matter how many times you do them. In fact, these traditional favorites often cause or aggravate lower back pain by pulling on the front of

the lower spine, which causes pelvic tilt. When this happens, your back is swayed inward and your lower abdomen pushes out. The posture you end up with only spotlights a potbelly appearance."[24]

Look at this headline from an article printed in The New York Times and other major publications.

Ab devices are little help in battle of bulge, study says

"A new study sponsored by the American Council on Exercise assessed the potential effectiveness of ab devices commonly marketed on TV infomercials. Dr. William Whiting, a specialist in biomechanics at California State University in Northridge, found no overall advantage to the devices, which cost from $75 to $120. Whiting and his collaborators concluded that crunches, whether done on one's own or aided by a device, do not use enough calories to result in weight loss and cannot 'spot reduce' accumulations of body fat. There was *no* apparent benefit or detriment to using popular abdominal exercise gadgets."[25]

It's secret time again!

You can have gorgeous abs and a strong trunk without doing situps or crunches or curling your spine!

In fact, you can achieve a beautiful torso with Oxycise! whether you're standing up, sitting, or lying down. Even if you have an injured back or spinal injuries, you can probably do this method. Oxycise! is an incredible tool in getting rid of fat in your torso area. Clients of mine have typically lost 2 to 4 inches per month from their waist while doing this method. Pretty exciting stuff! This includes clients from every level of fitness and mobility.

Here's how it works. You are about to learn the Oxycise! Basic Breath. After every inhale you will lift and tighten your abdominal area. As your diaphragm pushes down and your lower abdominal muscles lift up you essentially cause an internal isotonic exercise. In addition, you will learn to exhale with resistance which causes your abdominal muscles to flex involuntarily. All of this action in your torso creates a demand for oxygen in that area. Since you are providing plenty of oxygen, extra fat is easily metabolized and removed, your torso is trimmed and muscles are strengthened and toned. A wonderful side effect is that your back becomes straighter and stronger as your abdominal muscles increase their ability to support your spine.

One of my Oxycise! students had recently won a state body building championship and basically looked gorgeous from spending several hours a day in the gym. He tried this method exclusively for three weeks and tightened his abs 1½ inches! He claims that the toning he gets from 15 minutes of this method is equal to doing 400 crunches a day.

Another student, mother of two, with a severely damaged and painful back, was very disheartened with the extra weight she had accumulated and her inability to do traditional exercises.

She learned this method and lost 3 inches in three weeks. Needless to say, she was ecstatic. Some other side effects she shared with me were her ability to easily touch her toes, and she reported that her chiropractor had asked her what she was doing different in her life, because for the first time in years, her spine was aligned correctly.

Impressive, don't you think? I do. Be sure and let me know about your own impressive results.

Chapter Six

"Air Conditioning"

The Oxycise! Basic Breath

How do you breathe?

This is a test . . . .this is only a test.

1. Sit in a comfortable chair wearing loose-fitting clothing.
2. Put one hand on your stomach and one hand on your chest.
3. Blow all your air out (exhale).
4. Now suck air in (inhale).

Which way did your hands move during this test? The hand on your stomach should have pressed *in* toward your spine during the exhale and *out* during the inhale. Try it a few more times to be sure you feel it and are doing it correctly.

This is called:

Diaphragmatic Breathing

I'm assuming you know that your diaphragm doesn't breathe, but it is a muscle that contracts, creating a partial vacuum in the space between the lungs and the rib cage. As the air rushes in the abdomen pushes forward, which is the reason this is also called "abdominal breathing," but no air ever enters the abdomen. Your lungs are not muscles. They don't do anything by themselves. They only react to what's going on around them.

During the exhale, your diaphragm relaxes and returns to its gently arched resting shape.

Chest breathing.

Our society has become a bunch of chest breathers and hence suffers from numerous maladies including obesity, hyperventilation, and panic disorders.   Chest breathing means you only expand the rib cage during breathing. Even though it may look more dramatic, it is an inefficient form of breathing because only minimal air can enter and leave the lungs, which results in shallow and rapid breaths.

Now breathe.

Take a few more breaths now. Feel your ribs expand. Be sure to relax your shoulders — shoulders don't breathe.   Feel your abdomen expand. Close your eyes and feel the sensation of air filling your lungs clear down to the very bottom.

Doesn't that feel great?

It's time to get to work!   Just follow the step-by-step instructions at your own pace, and say goodby to fat.

Instructions for the Oxycise! Basic Breath

Inhale

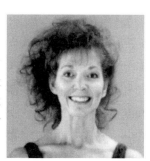

1.   *Inhale!* Breathe in quickly **through your nostrils**. Really burn it in. Air is cleansed and warmed as it enters through your nose. Remember the diaphragmatic breathing.

2. *Smile!* Pull the corners of your mouth back into a big smile while you inhale. It helps open the nostrils for better breathing, and it exercises and gives definition to your face muscles. But best of all, it's a reminder of how great you feel for taking control of your body.

3. *Relax!* Let your abdomen relax so you can take in as much air as possible.

Lift

1. *Lift!* After you've taken in all the oxygen you can, pull in and lift your lower abdomen.

2. *Tilt!* Tilt your pelvic area in and up. (Not out like a duck, but in like Elvis.)

3. *Squeeze!* Squeeze and lift your buttocks tightly.

4. *Squeeze!* Squeeze between your legs. (Kegel's exercise for ladies.)

Three Sniffs

1. *Sniff!* Take in three more sniffs of air. This works face, neck, and ab muscles, while ensuring full intake of oxygen.

Exhale

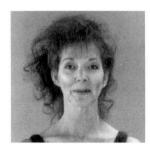

1. *Blow!* Form your lips like you're blowing through a straw (or playing a trumpet), making a small hole, and exhale with a lot of resistance. Feel your muscles right under your ribs. They should be taut.

2. *Head up!* Keep your head up. There's a real tendency to bend over while exhaling. Feel like there is a string keeping your head lifted.

3. *Buns tight!* Keep your buns tight from the "lift."

4. Force all air completely out.

Three Puffs

1. *Give three more puffs!* Try to force every bit of air out. (Remember to keep head up and buns tight.) This helps you make sure you're empty of air and increases your capacity to take in more oxygen. It also involuntarily works the abdominal muscles, adding tone and strength.

Oxycise!
Basic Breath Pattern

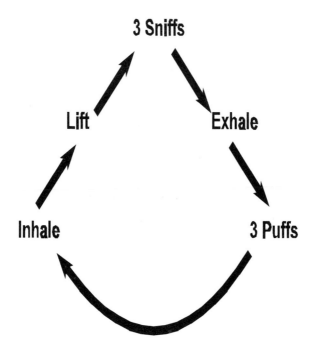

One Rep = Four Breath Patterns

Just complete the Basic Breath Pattern four times, and you've done one repetition ("rep") of the incredible Oxycise Basic Breath!

One Rep
of the
Oxycise! Basic Breath

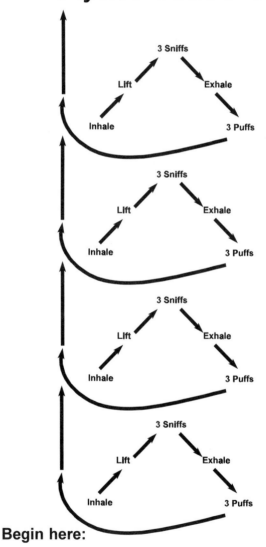

Begin here:

This simple process is the foundation of the entire Oxycise! program. Isn't it strange how things that are so easy, important, and effective get lost in our quest for the complex and dramatic?

Yes, it really is this simple to launch your metabolism to new heights. Every cell in your body will thank you, and before long your mirror will thank you also.

Ready to blast off???

Do one "rep" right now. Tap your fingers against your leg to keep track of the Four Basic Breath Patterns. Breathe deeply and with intensity. Can you feel your body waking up?

Chapter Seven

Level One

Workout

---

15 Minutes a Day
to
Self-Mastery

This day-by-day program is a suggested itinerary. It's okay to repeat a day, mix and match different positions, etc. Forget the "no pain, no gain" theory. There is *no impact* in any of these exercises, and you will not work up a heavy sweat.

Please use common sense as you stretch or flex muscles. It's great to increase your capacity but don't injure yourself.

15 minutes per day!

A full workout consists of only *30 Oxycise! reps per day!* Each rep takes about a half minute. That means that by doing 30 reps, you will only need to exercise **15 minutes per day!**

You may do more than 30 reps each day, and you will see astonishing results. Doing less than 30 reps per day, five or six days/week, however, will *not* give you the level of measurable results, that make this program so motivating.

More than once I've had participants who have learned Oxycise! call me and say in desperation, "Jill, you've got to help me! I'm just not losing weight." I then ask them to describe how frequently they Oxycise! *Without exception*, the answer will be, "I try to fit in a couple reps once in a while." Or even worse, "I don't Oxycise! but I'm trying to eat healthy." *You cannot just learn this information and expect it to take effect magically.* You do not have a magic body. Your body follows natural laws. You *must* increase your oxygen intake if you want to increase your metabolism. Oxycise! works. Oxygen is the key.

Now here's something exciting. Every single Oxycise! participant who truly follows the program has had 100% success. The phone calls and letters I receive are full of comments like:

> "I'm losing weight like crazy!"
> "I've never felt so good!"
> "My old pants fall off my hips!"
> "I've lost 4 inches from my waist!"
> "My body fat has gone down seven percent."

And I'll tell you something else exciting: Those 15 minutes do not need to be consecutive. So if you want to do 10 reps in the morning, 10 at lunchtime, and 10 in the evening, that's just fine. And if the phone rings or the baby cries, you can go take care of it and then return to finish your exercises.

Day 1

Learn the Oxycise! Basic Breath. Do it several times so it starts to become natural, and you don't have to look at the book to remember what to do.

Do one rep of the Oxycise! Basic Breath in each of the following positions. Complete this series a total of five times for today's workout of 30 Oxycise! reps.

1. Standing

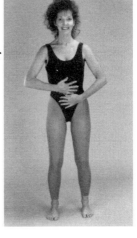

- Stand with feet about shoulder width apart.
- Keep head up.
- Tuck buns under.
- Bend knees.
- Use hands to press and lift abdomen.

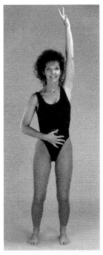

2. Overhead Reach — Right Arm

- Same body position as #1.
- Extend and stretch right arm above head.
- Keep hips pressing down.

3. Overhead Reach — Left Arm

- Same as #2, using left arm.

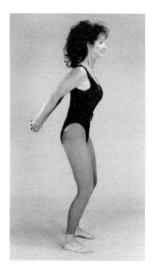

4. Shoulder Squeeze

- Same body position as #1.
- Grasp hands behind your back.
- Extend arms back.
- Squeeze shoulders back.

5. Rip the Floor

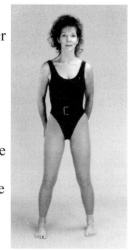

- Stand with feet about shoulder width apart.
- Bend knees slightly.
- "Rip" the floor apart. Grip with your feet and press out with your legs.
- Feel like you're trying to rip the floor apart, so that your outer calf and outer thigh muscles are tensed.
- Keep buns tight and maintain a pelvic tilt.

6. Pec Press

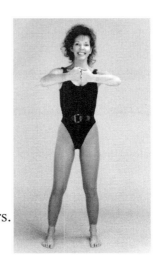

- Make hands into fists.
- Press knuckles together.
- Shape arms into an "O."
- Drop shoulders and keep head up.
- Press hard.
- Work the muscles in your pectorals, forceps, biceps, triceps, back, and shoulders.

Day 2

Congratulations! You are already on your second day. That's the beginning of a great habit!

Today you will learn four new positions. The Oxycise! Basic Breath should be easier to remember, so now you can start focusing on other parts of your body.

Flex your muscles.

Most of the positions require some muscle tension. Flexing muscles is an important aspect of Oxycise! and only you will know if you're flexing and stretching your muscles. The areas that you flex and stretch will demand oxygen. Remember what oxygen does for your body? It heals cells, builds cells, and *burns fat.* The Oxycise! Basic Breath done by itself will make a dramatic difference in your general health as well as increase your metabolism as you've already learned. By also stretching and flexing your muscles you will achieve a cardiovascular and resistance training workout at the same time! Check out the benefits you'll get by incorporating these isometric and isotonic positions. [26][27][28][29][30]

- Build lean body mass.
- Develop flexibility.
- Focus oxygen to that specific area.
- Reshape body.
- Lower blood pressure.
- Lower cholesterol.
- Reduce risk of diabetes.
- Reduce risk of heart disease.
- Strengthen musculo-skeletal system.
- Burn calories.
- Lose weight.
- Feel great!

Combining deep diaphragmatic breathing with these internal/external exercises is like giving your body a double whammy for great health!

Does the order of positions matter?

No. As you learn the new positions, insert them anywhere in the workout. If you like to be upright, then down on the floor, then on the chair, then upright, and so forth, you can arrange the order of the positions that way. If you like to do all the standing positions at one time, the sitting positions at one time, and end stretched out on the floor, that's fine too.

Add these four positions to the six from Day 1 to make a series of 10 Oxycise! reps. Complete this series three times for today's workout of 30 Oxycise! reps. Before you begin each Oxycise! Basic Breath, be sure your body is in proper position, flexed, and well aligned.

1. Squat

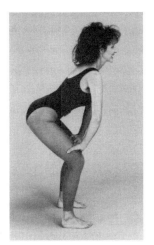

- Stick your rear end out. This is affectionately referred to as the "duck butt."
- Brace your feet and angle toes slightly inward.
- You should feel a stretch clear up over the ol' gluteus maximus and on your outer thighs.
- Place hands on legs and flex arms.

Off-the-Wall Series

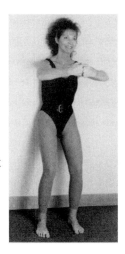

Use any wall in your house for support and/or resistance in this series of positions.

2. Lean and Press

- Stand with back pressed against the wall.
- Place feet a few inches out and press lower back against wall.
- Do a Pec Press with arms.

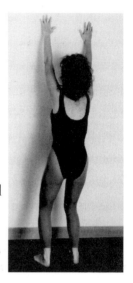

3. Sit and Stretch

- Face the wall and place both hands as high as you can.
- Sink down into a semi-sitting position.
- "Walk" your fingers up the wall to stretch a little farther with each inhale.
- Keep back aligned and head up.

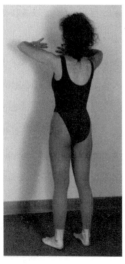

4. Wall Push Off

- Face wall and stand back a couple feet.
- Press hands into wall with elbows out.
- Lean forward keeping body and legs straight.
- Pelvic tilt, tighten buns.
- Keep heels on the floor.

Day 3 through Day 7

30 Oxycise! reps every day!

You now have a series of 10 Oxycise! reps you complete three times in order to do 30 Oxycise! reps for a daily workout. Do this workout every day this week. Use the charts to keep track of your progress.

At first it may take longer than 15 minutes because you're looking at pictures and figuring out how to place your body. But as you get the flow of Oxycise! you will be surprised how quickly you move through the positions.

Yes, it's really that simple!

Don't underestimate the power of Oxycise! just because it is so simple. Yes, it is a simple concept and it's simple to do. For those of you who think you can't achieve anything of worth unless it's complex, hang on. Work yourself up through all the Oxycise! levels and you will hit a level that will challenge your strength, flexibility, and coordination. However, *the higher levels are not necessary for weight loss and fat burning!*

Food power!

Be sure to fill your cells with the other nutrients they need. You're working hard to give them oxygen and to flush out toxins, so don't override any progress by dumping in garbage day after day.

During my years of battling with my body, I tried every food plan and chemical promise available. The *only* way to nourish your body for the long term so that you feel good and maintain your weight at a healthy level is to, once again, follow natural laws. Eat lots of fresh fruits, vegetables, whole grains, and other complex carbohydrates including rice, beans, corn, potatoes, whole wheat, pasta, and hearty breads.

Although these foods are readily available in a multitude of delicious variations, for many people it takes thought and effort to incorporate them fully into regular meals. For this reason I have written an easy-to-follow book called:

Fuel for Success!

The Food G.P.A. Plan introduced in *Fuel for Success!* is easy to follow and removes the feelings of "battle" and "deprivation" as you choose fuel for nutrition and enjoyment. I've also included lots of quick and easy meal ideas incorporating food items you are familiar with, but perhaps prepared in a different way. Mealtime actually becomes a pleasure rather than a hurdle.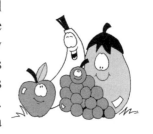

After eating this way for a few weeks, you will be amazed that you ever even craved some of the food you used to snarf down. In fact, it will often make you sick if you dive into rich or greasy food after having cleansed your body from the inside out.

Have a great week! You are on your way to health, vitality, and the body you deserve!

Week 2

Five new positions!

Each week for the next few weeks, you will add five new positions to your repertoire. Feel free to mix and match their order or to modify them if you have a physical limitation. For instance, if getting on your knees is a problem, then repeat another position, such as the Pec Press, instead.

Keep doing 30 Oxycise! reps per day, and you will love the changes happening to your body!

Hold-the-Bar Series

Hold to an exercise bar or the back of a chair.

1. Diagonal Leg Lift — Right Leg

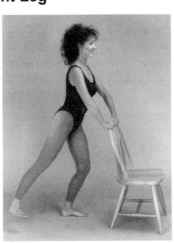

- Press arms in, against bar.
- Lift straight right leg to side and slightly back.
- Flex foot.
- Bend left leg.
- Pelvic tilt, tighten buns.
- Keep back and head aligned.

2. Diagonal Leg Lift — Left Leg

- Same as #1 using opposite legs.

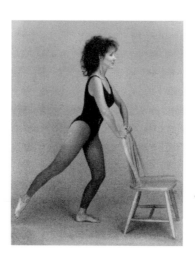

3. Bun Tuck — Right Leg

- Press arms in, against bar.
- Lift right leg straight to the back.
- Point toes.
- Bend left leg.
- Pelvic tilt, tighten buns.
- Keep back and head aligned.

4. Bun Tuck — Left Leg
- Same as #3, using opposite legs.

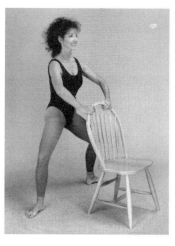

5. King Tut

- Spread feet with toes pointing out.
- Bend knees, keep knees directly over feet. (Be careful not to rotate knees forward.)
- Pelvic tilt, tighten buns.
- Press arms inward on bar.
- Keep back aligned and head up.
- Let torso sink, stretching inner thighs.

You now have a total of 15 Oxycise! Positions. Just complete this series twice for your daily total of 30 Oxycise! Reps.

Week 3

Chair Series

All five new positions for this week are done sitting on a chair. You now have a total of 20 Oxycise! positions. Just repeat any 10 positions for your daily total of 30 Oxycise! reps. Feel free to mix and match the positions in any order.

By the way, if there is a position that just doesn't work for you, just leave it out. There is not a single "magic" position that will trigger weight loss better than any other. *Breathing is the key!*

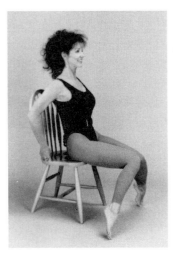

1. Sitting Knee Press

- Sit on front edge of chair.
- Lean back on hands, bend elbows.
- Pelvic tilt in, and tighten buns.
- Press knees together, feet out.

2. Inner Thigh Stretch

- Sit on front edge of chair.
- Keeping knees bent, spread legs, causing inner thigh stretch.
- Place hands on chair seat for support, squeeze shoulders back.
- Lean back slightly and keep body aligned.

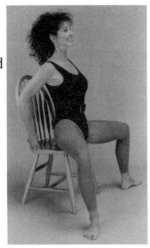

3. Sit 'n Twist — Right Arm Up

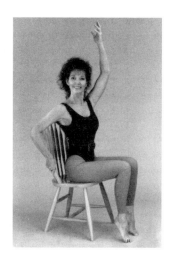

- Sit in middle of chair.
- Left hand grasp chair seat, pull up.
- Twist to left side.
- Right arm reach up and stretch.

4. Sit 'n Twist — Left Arm Up

- Same as #3, using opposite arms.

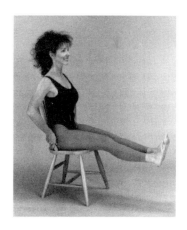

5. Double Leg Lift

- Sit back fully on chair.
- Support your back against chair back.
- Grasp both sides of chair seat and lift.
- Lift both legs.
- Flex feet.

Week 4

On-the-Floor Series I

All five new positions for this week are done on the floor. A carpeted living room or bedroom will work great, or you can use a rug, exercise mat, or towel to cushion a hard floor.

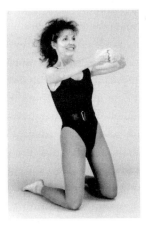

1. Kneeling Pec Press

- Kneel on carpet with knees slightly apart.
- Do a Pec Press with arms.
- Keep head up and body aligned.
- Pelvic tilt, tighten buns.
- Lean back slightly.

2. Sitting Butterfly

- Sit on the floor.
- Press feet together and pull toward torso.
- Press knees down for inner thigh stretch.
- Straighten back and keep head up.
- Grasp legs, ankles, or feet.
- Pull chest forward, "through" arms.

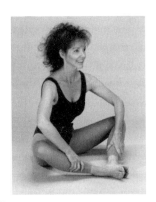

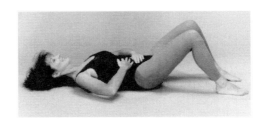

3. Basic Tilt

- Lie down on floor with knees bent.
- Pelvic tilt, tighten buns.
- Feel your abdomen "scoop" inward pressing down toward floor.

4. Knee Press

- Lie down on floor with knees bent.
- Press knees together, feet out.
- Pelvic tilt, tighten buns.
- Stretch arms above head with fingers interlocked.

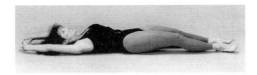

5. Torpedo One — Point Toes

- Lie down with legs extended.
- Stretch arms above head with fingers interlocked.
- Pelvic tilt, tighten buns.
- Tighten leg muscles, calves should pop up off floor.
- Point toes.

You've increased your repertoire up to 25 different positions. Repeat any five of the positions to add up to your daily total of 30 Oxycise! reps.

Hit the mall!

I'll bet you're feeling great these days. Inches and pounds have started to come off. As soon as your clothes start to feel a little loose, treat yourself to a shopping trip and spend some time looking for a pair of pants or other item that accentuates your best features.

As you shed sizes, it is important to reinforce your positive changes. Don't wait until you've reached your end goal to improve your wardrobe. Set short-term goals like "I will treat myself to a new outfit with every inch lost from my hips (every 10 pounds lost, every month I Oxycise! regularly, etc.)." It will be exciting as the dressing room mirror ceases to be your enemy and becomes your good friend!

Week 5

Smooth Transition Between Positions!

Keep working on having a smooth transition between positions. Yes, it's okay to stop between positions, but it makes for a fast workout if you move directly into the next one. As you do your final exhale of each Oxycise! rep, move your body into the next position.

On the Floor Series II

Once again you get to exercise lying down. Don't you love it?

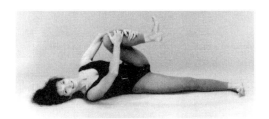

1. Knee Hug — Right Leg

- Lie slightly on left side.
- Pull right knee in toward chest.
- Force lower leg out against hands.
- Extend left leg and tighten muscles.
- Flex feet.

2. Knee Hug — Left Leg
- Same as #1 using opposite legs.

3. Back Leg Lift — Right Leg
- Roll on left side toward stomach.
- Lift right leg up and back.
- Press hands on floor.
- Lift head.
- Point toes.

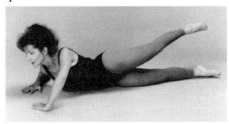

4. Back Leg Lift — Left Leg
- Same as #3, using opposite legs and arms.

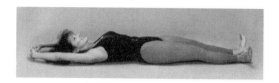

5. Torpedo Two — Flex Feet
- Same as Torpedo One, except for flexed toes.

You've done it!
You now know 30 Oxycise! positions.

Increase intensity!

Increase your intensity every day and you will be surprised at your improved strength and endurance. Doesn't it feel great to have control of your body?

End of Level One!

Pat yourself on the back! You've been working hard to learn something new, and you've stuck with it. *That's fantastic!* Old habits are hard to change.

Is there more to learn?

There is always more to learn, *but* you don't need to proceed to the higher Oxycise! levels to lose weight. So if you have these patterns memorized and don't want to learn any more, that's just fine. Your body will continue to thank you for the increased oxygen capacity you are developing.

Level 2 and each of the more advanced videos listed at the beginning of this book will introduce new routines that will develop strength, range of motion, and flexibility -- as well as add variety to your daily routine. Each consecutive level becomes more challenging and you should continue to breathe with lots of gusto and power, but again, the higher levels are not necessary for weight loss!

Keep on breathin'!

Besides your regular workout session, take advantage of those extra minutes you have each day and do some extra Oxycise! reps. Try them while you are: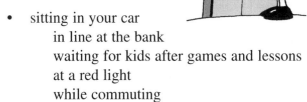

- sitting in your car
    in line at the bank
    waiting for kids after games and lessons
    at a red light
    while commuting
- in your kitchen
    waiting for the beeper on the microwave
    standing at the stove
    waiting for "Junior" to finish his cereal
- during commercials while watching TV
- waiting for the elevator
- waiting in line at the grocery store
- during a boring meeting
- waiting for a computer program to load

Get the idea? Every one of us has countless "extra" minutes each day where we can fit in a few more productive breaths.

Have fun with Oxycise! and be sure to write/call/email (my address is in the front and back of this book) to let me know of your experiences and discoveries as you take control of your body from the inside out!

Suggested Level One: 15-Minute Workout Order

Standing

1. Standing
2. Overhead Reach — Right Arm
3. Overhead Reach — Left Arm
4. Shoulder Squeeze
5. Squat
6. Pec Press
7. Rip the Floor

Hold-the-Bar Series

8. Diagonal Leg Lift — Right Leg
9. Bun Tuck — Right Leg
10. Diagonal Leg Lift — Left Leg
11. Bun Tuck — Left Leg
12. King Tut

Chair Series

13. Knee Press
14. Inner Thigh Stretch
15. Sit 'n Twist — Right Arm Up

16. Sit 'n Twist — Left Arm Up
17. Double Leg Lift

Off-the-Wall Series

18. Lean and Press
19. Sit and Stretch
20. Wall Press

On-the-Floor Series

21. Kneeling Pec Press
22. Sitting Butterfly
23. Basic Tilt
24. Knee Press
25. Knee Hug — Right Leg
26. Back Leg Lift — Right Leg
27. Knee Hug — Left Leg
28. Back Leg Lift — Left Leg
29. Torpedo One — Point Toes
30. Torpedo Two — Flex Toes

Part Three

You Can
Do It!

**"There is nothing impossible
to him who will try."**

Alexander the Great

Chapter Eight

Your Set Point
You CAN Control It

According to theory, your body determines the weight at which it can best survive and then tenaciously defends that weight to the best of its ability. This has come to be commonly known and referred to as your set point weight. This means that if you diet to lose weight, you will gain back the weight. The reverse is also true. If you are force fed to gain weight, you will lose the weight when you are allowed to eat normally.

Let's suppose you think you need to lose a few pounds and so you put yourself on a diet program. You proceed to keep your body from receiving the calories and nutrients it is used to and needs to maintain its current set point weight. You will initially lose weight. But your body doesn't know the difference between a "self-imposed" restriction and a "lost-in-the-desert" forced starvation, so it reacts the same in both situations. As you deprive yourself, your body will start to conserve energy in every way it can because it doesn't know how long this disaster is going to last. Your fat-storing enzymes will increase and your fat-burning enzymes decrease — you need to hang on to those fat stores as long as possible so you can make it through the current "famine." Your muscle tissue is also decreased and you become lethargic, cranky, and out of energy.

Remember that you have a magnificent body. It will not sit passively and starve to death — it will first put up a fight. When humans are without proper nourishment, we will eat things we normally would never even consider. Consider the experiences of prisoners of war or those who have been in concentration camps.

Some years ago I participated in wilderness survival programs in the deserts of southern Utah. These programs each lasted for only one month and basic flour, rice, a few vegetables, salt, and water were provided. However, within a couple weeks of each program, I saw regular college students from middle income families pick up live ants from the ground and eat them. They went in streams and ate the bugs from the underside of the wet rocks. They fried maggots after collecting them from cattails. They were given a sheep and not only did they eat all the regular meat, but also finished off anything they could chew, including the stomach, intestines and other innards, ending with the brains and eyeballs. My point in describing this is to emphasize the point that your body will take over and eat anything in its efforts to survive if you put it in a position that deprives it of its regular nourishment.

If within a few weeks of a wilderness survival program, people are willing to eat the kinds of things I just mentioned, what do you think will happen if you deprive your body of nutrients and yet still have a pantry and freezer full of all kinds of delicious foods? There is virtually no hope of permanently maintaining that regimen.

Now here's the kicker. Because your body is so smart, once it is able to start making up for its deprivation, it's going to make darn sure it's ready for the next "famine". So besides gaining back all the weight you lost through your diet, you get a few extra pounds thrown in for protection. Not only that, but your metabolism stays at a decreased level and your set point weight just went up a few more pounds. The next time you diet, your body will be trying to defend the higher set point and the cycle continues as your body gets smarter and stores more fat for the next disaster.

The set point mechanism has also been described as a "thermostat" such as you have in your home to control the heating or cooling. Most of the body's functions operate on such a principle.

Here are a few examples:

Sugar levels in the blood. When something happens to raise or lower those levels, the body makes adjustments to bring the sugar levels back into the normal range.

PH balance of the blood. This keeps your body from becoming too acidic or alkaline.

Oxygen. Say you're calmly walking to the bus stop, and then you look up and see the bus is about to leave and so you suddenly sprint a whole block, running and waving your arms. You barely catch the bus and get a seat. Your muscle cells were required to burn large quantities of oxygen to support your running and now the oxygen content of the muscles is below your set point for oxygen and there is an oxygen debt. That gap must be filled in order for you to be comfortable, in fact it must be filled in order for you to survive. So what do you do once you get on the bus? You "binge" on oxygen. You gasp or pant until the gap has been filled and the oxygen debt has been repaid and your breathing rate returns to normal.

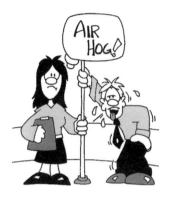

Has anyone ever accused you of "overbreathing" after running or climbing stairs?

Body temperature. You get goose bumps when it's cold and sweat when it's hot — all because you have a set point or "thermostat" for body temperature. You may get a fever when your body is trying to fight a foreign organism, meaning that your body temperature set point has moved higher. This set point is very much like the body weight set point. Once you take away the cause of the fever (the reason the body temperature set point is high), the body temperature set point will be reset to a lower temperature. Likewise, if you take away the cause of the body weight set point being high, it will reset itself to a lower set point.

Body weight. The organ that regulates your body weight is called the hypothalamus. It is an important organ in the central nervous system located at the base of the brain. It will regulate your body weight according to *its* perception of what you need at any given time.[31]

So how do you influence your hypothalamus to reset your set point to a lower body weight? This is the key to successful, permanent, and healthy weight loss. By first identifying the opposite process — how to raise your set point, maybe you can better understand how to lower it.

How to *raise* your set point:

- Breathe shallowly.
- Yo-yo dieting — especially effective.
- Eat high fat diets.
- Eat high sugar diets.
- Sit around a lot.
- Go on deprivation diets.

The all-too-typical American lifestyle.

How to *lower* your set point:

- Breathe deeply.
- Increase your oxygen consumption.
- Eat low-fat, fresh, oxygen-rich food.
- Eat when you need food.
- Live an active life.

The Oxycise! lifestyle.

Oxycise! and healthy eating are natural ways to influence your hypothalamus to lower your set point. As you eat life-giving food, your body will feel satisfied and quit hoarding stores of fat for emergencies. You are now providing yourself with the nutrients you need, so your body willingly gives up its extra fat stores. As you breathe in extra oxygen while flexing and stretching your muscles, your body will respond immediately by flushing out excess fat and other toxins.

An incredible result of living the Oxycise! lifestyle is that you will remove the cause of your set point being too high. With Oxycise! your set point will naturally be lowered until you reach the body size you should be. Once you have achieved your optimum size to maintain good health, your set point will no longer drop, since to lose too much weight would be potentially harmful.

If you've been overweight for much of your life, you will thrill in lowering your set point. As you follow the Oxycise! principles, you will be surprised at how painless the process is. Yes, it does take some time — 15 minutes a day — and some effort to learn new habits, but the results are so motivating and the freedom from obesity is true nirvana. You're gonna love it!!!

Yes, with Oxycise! you *can and will* lower your set point permanently!

Chapter Nine

Keep the Score,
Know the Score,
and the Score Will Improve!

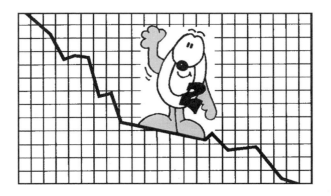

To weigh or not to weigh.

I recently was talking with the fitness director of an expensive health spa. When she found out that I regularly have clients weigh and measure their bodies, she responded, "Oh, I've spent years trying to get our clients to throw away their scales!" Their emphasis was on trying to help people just feel good about themselves.

At another elite health/weight loss spa I visited, the program director told me, "We never have our guests weigh themselves after they've been here for a week, because the results are too discouraging. Some even gain weight."

Now I ask you,

"How can you make a needed change in your life without tracking progress?"

"How can you pay $2,000 to stay at a weight loss facility for a week and go home without measuring and achieving progress?"

Something's wrong here.

When I was in high school, I drove an old car that had a broken gas gauge. Rather than fix it, I drove by "feel." I tried to "feel" if it was about time to fill it up with fuel or not. Needless to say, I was late for class, I was late for work, I hitchhiked to gas stations, I had to push it out of the middle of the road, and otherwise waste my time and miss opportunities — all because I didn't measure my progress.

Keep the score,
know the score,
and the score will improve!

This is critical! If your "score" is already where you want it, then you don't need to pay attention to any of what I'm saying. This is for those of you who really want to improve your score.

I have never seen anyone make permanent body changes without:

1. Setting specific goals.
2. Tracking progress.

How much should you weigh?

There is no absolute answer for everyone. The variety in our body shapes adds beauty and interest to our world.

Here are some guidelines to help you:

1. Do not try to look like models or actors. In order to have your body featured on the front of magazines, you have to devote your entire life to achieving that look. Many times, if not most of the time, it's only achievable at the expense of true health. You have a life. Let your body serve you rather than you being a slave to it.

2. Use the standard Metropolitan Life Insurance Height and Weight chart for a general idea of where you should be. (See the book Chart Your Success.) I can't tell you how many times, during the years I was overweight, that I had people tell me, "You're not fat, you're just big boned." So I tried to believe them, but I knew my body didn't feel good the way it was.

An amazing thing happened when I made my major body change several years ago. Nobody tells me I have big bones anymore. In fact, now I hear things like, "You have small bones," "Your shoulders are so narrow," "Your rib cage is so small." Did my bones change that much? No, of course not. I just got rid of all the layers of fat surrounding my bone structure.

My point in sharing that experience is to encourage you to be realistic when you look at the chart and are trying to determine if you should be at the lower or higher end of the weight range for your height. You'll notice there is quite a spread in weight for any given height. Physicians use a caliper to measure the bones on the side of your elbow to determine your frame size. In Chart Your Success I have described how to measure yourself at home. Your elbow measurement will give you a general idea of which end of the weight chart spread you should be.

When all things are considered, you know if you feel good at your weight.

3. *Remember a former time when you loved your body.* For people like me, we never had a time like that. So when setting a weight goal I had to do a little experimenting. But for many people, there has been a time in your *adult* life when you felt healthy and liked the way your clothes fit. (Please don't get distorted with this and try to fit in the same size you did when you were in 6th grade.)

Visualize yourself as you were then. Bring back those healthy thoughts and attitudes toward yourself.

Set a goal and tell everyone about it.

Take a few minutes to think about what you really want to accomplish. Remember that goals are stars to help guide you, not sticks with which to beat yourself.

Write it down. *A goal not written is only a wish.* Be specific so you have a way to track progress and be accountable to yourself.

Tell everyone what you're doing. This will make you accountable to others besides yourself. Also, you will be amazed at the support friends and family can provide when you're feeling discouraged.

**Weigh
and
measure
regularly.**

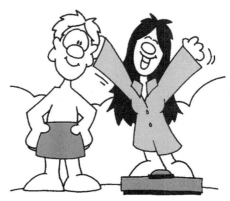

1.   Start right now. There's no time like the present, so turn to the Chart Your Success and grab a pencil and a tape measure. Write down the date. Weigh yourself. Measure the body areas you want to track.

2.   Weigh every morning. I recommend weighing yourself every morning, and writing it down. You will not show a steady weight loss every single day! Your body is not a machine. If you understand and accept that, then you are farther down the road to success. There are many reasons for the fluctuations you see on the scale such as menstrual cycle, late-night eating, and normal body processes. As you track your weight each day, you will become used to these fluctuations.

3.   Measure once a week. You can measure every day if you want, but it's a little more time consuming than weighing, which is why I suggest doing it weekly. Your records will be more consistent if you measure without any clothes on.

Measure the places you're interested in tracking, but for most men, a waist and chest measurement are sufficient. For women, rib cage, waist, hips, and one thigh are plenty to keep track of. You can assume that if these areas are firming up, the rest of your body is also.

4. Use Chart Your Success. This book is for your use. Modify the charts if you prefer to keep records in a different manner, but keep the score. As you progress, it will be gratifying and motivating to look back and see how far you've come.

What about body fat percentage?

As I've initially weighed and measured clients in both private consultations and workshop situations, nothing brings a groan of despair more often than the anticipation of their body fat measurement. If this number is high, you can no longer pretend that the high numbers on your scale are because of all your lean muscle mass.

Why should you care what your body fat percentage is? Because numerous studies have shown that body fat percentage has a significant correlation to both health and long life. For example, the Framingham studies of the National Institutes of Health provide convincing evidence that high body fat significantly increases the risk of heart attacks, strokes, and even some types of cancer.[32]

Let's start with dispelling some common myths about body fat:

Myth #1
It usually takes several weeks of rigorous diet and exercise before realizing any change in body fat.

> **Absolutely not!** With Oxycise! you can measure a change within the first two weeks (usually the first week).

Myth #2
The most fat loss you can expect to lose each month is a half percent.

> **Absolutely not!** With Oxycise! participants commonly reduce their body fat percentage by 3% to 4% the first month. Reducing it by 5% to 10% within the first two months is very attainable by those who live the Oxycise! lifestyle. It will continue to improve according to your body's needs until you arrive in the "Excellent" category on the Body Fat Chart. (See Chart Your Success.)

Myth #3
If your body fat is in the "Excellent" category, you won't have any soft spots.

> **Absolutely not!** Especially with women. You are supposed to have some fat, and if you don't have enough then your body won't function well. If you are a 40- year-old woman weighing 130 pounds, with 20% body fat, that means that you have 26 pounds of fat on your body. Some of the 26 pounds

of fat is around the intestines, under your skin, and in each breast, but you are designed to carry some around your hips and thighs, too. Women are supposed to have curves. With Oxycise! you'll get rid of the rolls and dimples, leaving the curves the way they were meant to be.

Obesity, according to definition, exists when more than 20% of body weight is composed of fat in men and 25% or more in women.[33] Have your body fat tested by your doctor or at a local health club.

Don't get upset if your body fat percentage is high. You now have the means to effect a permanent change. Oxycise! burns fat and builds lean body mass. Go have your body fat rechecked in a month or two. Refer to the Body Fat Percentage Table in Charts for Success to track your progress.

You will be amazed at the rapid improvement of your body fat measurement as you incorporate the simple and basic principles of Oxycise! into your life!

What is Body Mass Index?

Body Mass Index (BMI) is quickly becoming the standard way of talking about obesity, since it is an easy way to compare the fatness of people of different heights. BMI is a ratio of body weight to height and is calculated as weight in kilograms divided by height in meters squared.[34] To figure yours, you can follow the formula at the end of this section.

Federal guidelines suggest that people should keep their body mass indexes under 25. Anything more than that is too much, and over 27 is considered obese.[35] The National

Health and Nutrition Examination Survey, conducted on 30,000 people between 1991 and 1994, shows that 59 percent of U.S. men and 49 percent of women have BMIs over 25. The survey also found that people in their 50s are the fattest with 73 percent of men and 64 percent of women this age having BMIs over 25.[36]

This means that millions and millions of people in our country are overweight. Fortunately for you, you now have correct principles to apply in your life, and you will no longer be part of those statistics.

How to Figure Your BMI

Weight in pounds x .45 = Weight in kilograms

Height in inches   x .0254 = Height in meters

Height in meters   x Height in meters = Height in meters squared

Weight in kg   ÷ Height in meters squared = BMI

You will find BMI worksheets in Chart Your Success to help you figure and keep track of your own BMI. Body Mass Index is a good way for you to identify if your weight puts you at risk for health problems. A common sense exception to this method would be those who are in heavy weight-training programs and have extremely dense muscle mass. In those cases, a body fat measurement would be more accurate.

Example BMI Measurement

A 5 feet 10 inches tall man who weighs 193 pounds.

193 pounds	x .45	=	86.85 kg
70 inches	x .0254	=	1.78 meters
1.78 m	x 1.78 m	=	3.17 m
86.85 kg	÷ 3.17	=	27.4 BMI

Do not put value judgments on your weight or measurements.

You do not have a "good" day because you lost a pound, and you do not have a "bad" day because your weight is up a pound! You are not a success in life if your body fat or your BMI are low; you are not a failure in life if your body fat or BMI are high! You are only keeping score so you will know the score and can take the steps to improve the score.

You have a "good" day and a great life as you make daily decisions to live a healthy lifestyle.

Chapter Ten

Yes!

You Can Master

Your Body

from the

Inside Out!

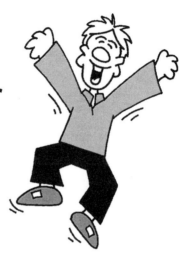

Congratulations!

You have arrived at the conclusion of this course and are ready to proceed with the most exciting adventure of your life . . . an adventure that will bring you a body of health and a life of freedom that you have never felt before. It also happens to be an adventure that will make you slender.

In Chapter One you learned the most common mistakes people make in weight loss efforts. You don't want to waste any more of your valuable time, money, and energy on mistakes. So review the "17 Avoidable Mistakes" with pen in hand and commit to never making these errors.

Avoidable Mistake #1

You are following the wrong "road map."

Now commit!

❏   I truly want to change my life. I won't confuse mere action with correct action.

Avoidable Mistake #2

You treat your body like a machine instead of like the incredible natural creation it truly is.

Now commit!

❏   Never again will I go against the laws of nature as I care for my body. I will feed it plenty of oxygen and good food. I will stop dumping unnecessary chemicals into my body.

Avoidable Mistake #3

You think your body has let you down and is not responding to your good care.

Now commit!

❏   I won't blame or give up on my body just because it has been responding in the best way it could considering all the stupid things I've put it through. I will make Oxycise! part of my life so that rather than barely surviving, my body may begin to *thrive!*

Avoidable Mistake #4

You use/consider food and sedentary living as rewards.

Now commit!

❑ There are times when I and those around me deserve recognition and rewards. I will choose those rewards that are healthy, motivating, and rejuvenating.

Avoidable Mistake #5
You embrace the Scarcity Mentality instead of the Abundance Mentality.

Now commit!

❑ Living a healthy lifestyle only deprives me of poor health, lethargy, and fat. I will actively seek an abundant life with true benefits.

Avoidable Mistake #6
You're in search of the "quick fix" and "instant remedy."

Now commit!

❑ I will immediately stop searching for instant, no effort remedies for my weight and health problems. I will learn to harness my body's natural power to achieve a healthy weight and lifestyle.

Avoidable Mistake #7
Your mind has been imprinted with the need to diet.

Now commit!

❑ I will never, ever, ever restrict my calorie intake through diet, starvation, appetite suppressants, surgery, or any other method. I now understand how destructive these methods are and I am seeking long term health, vitality, and joyful living.

Avoidable Mistake #8

You've been misled into believing that bouncing, shaking and sweating are the best ways to lose weight.

Now commit!

❑   I understand that oxygen is the key to boosting my metabolism. I can increase my oxygen consumption right in the privacy of my home without injuring muscles, joints, or bones. Never again will I neglect my body's needs because I don't like to bounce, shake, and sweat.

Avoidable Mistake #9

You've been sucked into trying to look like what the media presents as normal and healthy.

Now commit!

❑   I have a life. I will not be a slave to the media-influenced perception that I should be skinnier than is healthy for my body.

Avoidable Mistake #10

You don't have time to work out.

Now commit!

❑   I now know that all I need is a small amount of the right kind of exercise. I will commit to 15 minutes of Oxycise! each day.

Avoidable Mistake #11

You don't want to spend hours reading treatises on

exercise physiology.
Now commit!

❑   If reading all the explanations of how the body works becomes burdensome, I will skip to the video program and begin the practical application.

Avoidable Mistake #12
You don't want to change any habits.

Now commit!

❑   I will make the effort necessary to liftoff from the gravity pull of mistaken habits that are keeping me overweight and unhealthy and enter the Oxycise! orbit for a slender, healthy life.

Avoidable Mistake #13
You are a shallow chest breather.

Now commit!

❑   I want to provide my body with the oxygen it needs to be healthy and slim. I will learn diaphragmatic breathing and make it a way of life.

Avoidable Mistake #14
You live in a push-button society.

Now commit!

❑   I will continue to enjoy the conveniences of modern society, but I will not neglect my body at the same time. I will consciously breathe more deeply and fully every day of my life, applying the methods and principles of Oxycise!

Avoidable Mistake #15
Stress has literally "taken your breath away."

Now commit!

❑   I will remember to breathe deeply and well in times of stress so my body will be in a better position to handle external pressures.

Avoidable Mistake #16
You don't eat oxygen rich food.

Now commit!

❑   I respect my body and will not stuff it with the garbage food that is available today. I will make fresh, live, oxygen-rich food the bulk of my food intake.

Avoidable Mistake #17
You don't Oxycise!

Now commit!

❑   I will Oxycise!

You now have all the tools.

Now you have just what you need to accomplish your objectives with your body shape, size, and health. You have learned to provide your body with enough oxygen for each cell to be able to function at an optimum level. You have learned to harness your body's natural power to cleanse itself and to maintain the appropriate amount of body fat. You have discovered that you can accomplish these things in a minimal amount of time. You also have learned the Oxycise! Level One 15-Minute Workout so you can apply your new knowledge and achieve the results you desire.

Our paths need not part here. I have been with you this far, and I wish to be with you as you continue on your adventure. Let me know of any discoveries you make while doing Oxycise! Many participants have discovered improvements for the breathing pattern, body positions, or nutrition plan that have been incorporated into the current book. I appreciate those of you who are willing to share your discoveries. Nothing would please me more than to learn new things from you. I commend you for your determination to find truth and apply it in your life. I look forward to hearing from you.

Oxycise! is powerful. It makes common sense, it feels good, and *it works!* You *can* unlock your tremendous mental and physical powers to solve the chronic underlying problems of poor health and excess weight. You *will* focus on these true principles that bring you the freedom of health, fitness, and joyful living.

Yes! You can have the body you want and deserve with Oxycise!

You have the power. It is already within you.

> **"What lies behind us and what lies before us are tiny matters compared to what lies within us."**
>
> **Oliver Wendell Holmes**

REFERENCES

[1]Sorenson, M. *MegaHealth*. National Institute of Fitness, 1991, pp. 19-22.

[2]Gutfield, G. Flex down hypertension: simple exercise drops blood pressure in minutes. *Prevention*, March 1993, v45, n3, p. 12(2).

[3]Covey, S. *The 7 Habits of Highly Effective People*, Simon & Schuster, New York, 1989, p. 219.

[4]Sorenson, M. *MegaHealth*. National Institute of Fitness, 1991, pp. 13, 17.

[5]Schneider, K. Mission Impossible. *People*, June 3, 1996, v45, pp. 65-74.

[6]Fried, R., *Breath Connection*. Insight Books, 1990, p. 182.

[7]Mannerberg, D. *Aerobic Nutrition*. Hawthorn/Dutton, New York, 1988, p. 37.

[8]Mannerberg, D. *Aerobic Nutrition*, Hawthorn/Dutton, New York, 1988, p. 38.

[9]Baker, E. *The Unmedical Miracle: Oxygen*. Drelwood Communications, 1991, p. 80.

[10]Baker, E. *The Unmedical Miracle: Oxygen*. Drelwood Communications, 1991, pp. 31-32.

[11]Girandola, R., Ph.D. author interview, May 28, 1998.

[12]Akers, M., author interview, June 18, 1998.

[13]Fried, R. *Breath Connection*, Insight Books, 1990, p. 63.

[14] Fried, R. *Breath Connection*, Insight Books, 1990, pp. 151, 158.

[15]Baker, E. Oxygen: the key to energy. *Total Health*, Oct. 1991, p. 18(2).

[16]Guyton, A. MD. *Function of the Human Body*. W.B. Saunders Co., Philadelphia, 1975, p. 4.

[17]Shields, J. Lymph, lymph glands, and homeostasis. *Lymphology*, v25, n4, Dec. 1992, pp. 147-153.

[18]Best, C.H.; Taylor, N.B. *The Human Body.* Henry Holt and Co., New York.

[19]Sparkman, D. Anabolic signals: cell hydration for proper protein synthesis. *Muscle & Fitness*, Jan. 1994, v55, n1, p. 58(4)

[20]Asimov, I. *On the Human Body*. Bonanza Books, New York, 1985.

[21]Carlson, A., et. al. *The Machinery of the Body.* University of Chicago Press, 1972.

[22]Dunham, R. New options in oxygen therapy: Can an increase in oxygen reverse a disease process? *Independent Living*, Nov.-Dec. 1990, v5, n4, p. 61(2).

[23]Hill, J., MD. CU Medical Research, author interview, April 1996.

[24]Cooper, R. *Low Fat Living*. Rodale Press, Emmaus, Pennsylvania, 1996, p. 162.

[25]Brody, J. "Ab" devices are little help in battle of bulge, study says. *The Denver Post*, Wed. Jan. 8, 1997, p. 6A.

[26]Baker, J. Resistance training basics. *American Fitness*, May-June 1994, p. 26.

[27]Boyden, R. Resistance exercise training is associated with decreases in serum low-density lipoprotein cholesterol levels in premenopausal women. Health Index.

[28]Dunham, R. New options in oxygen therapy: Can an increase in oxygen reverse a disease process? *Independent Living*, Nov.-Dec. 1990, v5, n4, p. 61(2).

[29]Gutfield, G. Muscle up your metabolism. *Prevention*, Aug. 1991, p. 60(6).

[30]Medical Update. Medical Education and Research Foundation, Oct. 1993, p. 3.

[31]Sorenson, M. *MegaHealth*. National Institute of Fitness, 1991, pp. 49-65.

[32]Futrex — 1000 Bodyfat Tester. User's Manual, Version 2.0, pp. 1, 15.

[33]Obesity. Grolier Multimedia Encyclopedia. Version 7.05, 1995.

[34]Body Mass Index. Grolier Multimedia Encyclopedia. Version 7.05, 1995.

[35]Meckler, L. Doctors get guides on treating obesity. *The Denver Post*, Wed. Oct. 30, 1996, p. 12A.

[36]Associated Press. Scales tipped: Most people overweight. *The Des Moines Register*, Wed. Oct. 16, 1996, p. 4A.

About the Author

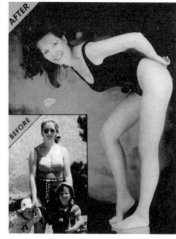

Jill R Johnson is the owner of Oxycise! International, Inc. and has dedicated more than 10 years to the development of The Oxycise! System. Having conquered her own struggles with being overweight for much of her life, she knows first hand the social, emotional, and physical challenges required to make lifestyle changes.

Jill is a vibrant and energetic educator, seminar and workshop leader, and author, and has been featured on many television and radio shows throughout the United States and Canada. Her seminars and classes are presented with energy, humor, and warmth, as she not only teaches techniques, but lays the groundwork for each individual to take control of their personal health and fitness.

She is delightfully living her dream with her husband and four children in the beautiful Rocky Mountains of Colorado.

I wish you the best
in your personal endeavors.
Remember,
You have the power!

Oxycise! International, Inc. continues to consult individuals, groups and businesses who want to take control of their body weight, health, and fitness. To obtain additional Oxycise! System information, please contact:

Oxycise! International, Inc.
8170 S. University Blvd., #110
Littleton, CO 80122

(303)224-9588
www.oxycise.com